AF364648

CREATE HEALTH WITH YOUR SEXUAL ENERGY

IRÉNE ANDERSSON

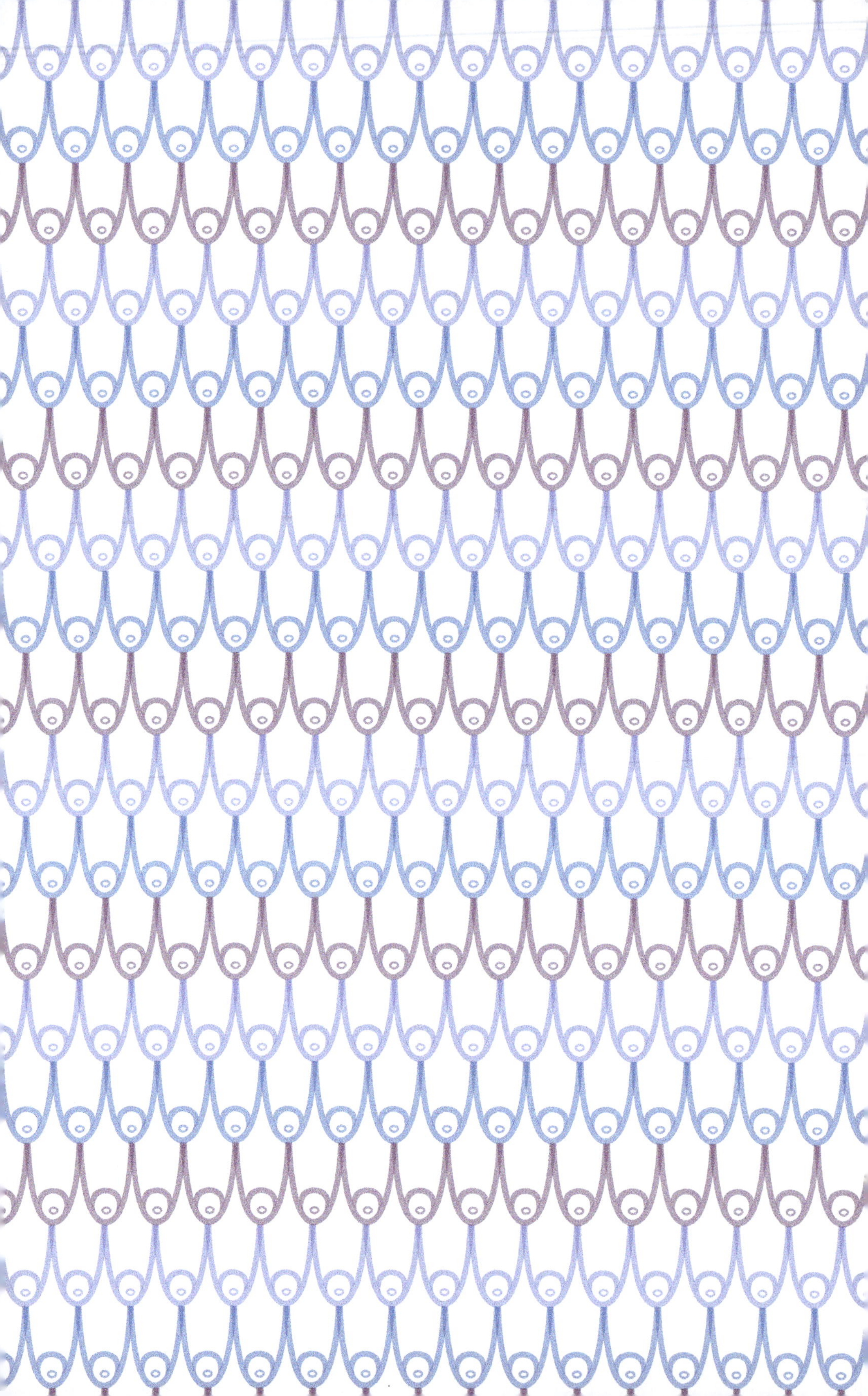

CREATE HEALTH
with your
SEXUAL ENERGY

The Tao Approach to Men's Well-Being

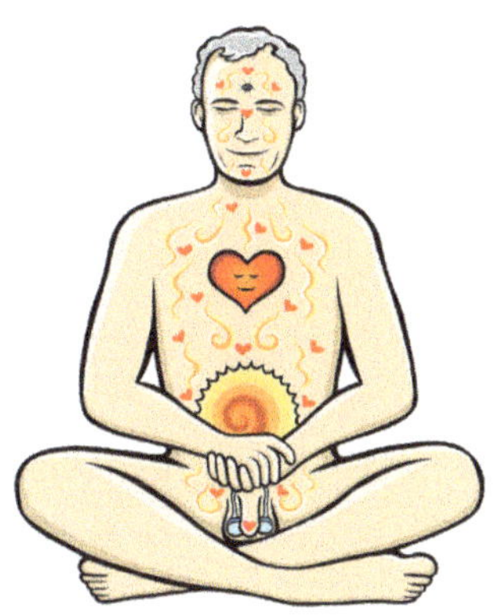

Illustrations: Lisa C. Larsson
Translation: Johan Badh

IRÉNE ANDERSSON

Also by the author:

Create Health with Your Sexual Energy: The Tao Approach to Women's Well-Being, 2020

Create Health with Your Sexual Energy: The Tao Approach to Men's Well-Being

© Iréne Andersson. Procreative AB, Stockholm, 2020.
www.bodycoach.nu
www.pelvicfloorawareness.com

Original title: Mannens Tao: Vägen till lycka, potens och livskraft!
© Iréne Andersson. Stockholm, Sweden 2014.
Publisher: ProCreative AB

The reproduction of the contents of this book, in whole or in part, without the consent of the author, is prohibited by the copyright law. This applies to text as well as illustrations.

The author does not provide any medical advice or prescribe the use of any exercise as a treatment for any disorder, and does not take responsibility for possible injuries while performing these exercises. As always, wrong practice, as well as inaccurate or inadequate exercise, can cause unwanted effects to some people. In case of ailments, pain or insecurity, it is recommended to seek professional help. The exercises are also not intended to cure disease, but are designed to create opportunities for recovery, self-awareness and development.

Tao is spelled Tao according to Wales-Giles, which created a method of transliterating Chinese characters into the Latin alphabet. The method was developed during the 19th century, but is often replaced by the pinyin method, and Tao is then spelled Dao. In this text, the spelling Tao is generally used, except in some Chinese book titles.

Text: Iréne Andersson
Illustrations: Lisa C. Larsson, www.tecknarlisa.com
Layout & cover: Ann-Sofie Hammarström, www.lillablatornet.se
Translation: Johan Badh

ISBN 978-91-981931-5-2   P o D
ISBN 978-91-981931-4-5   e-book

Praise for *"Create Health with Your Sexual Energy"*

The Taoist alchemical spiritual tradition is closest to my heart. It's been my experience over the last 35 years of personal practice that each of us will never embody our true spirituality without first embracing and making conscious our sexual energy. Every human being who is born on this planet will have to navigate this journey. Some will do it unconsciously with much frustration and pain, and others will be blessed to find a modern Taoist alchemist who can clarify and simplify the terrain in everyday language.

I highly recommend these books written by someone who has taken this journey herself and made it her life's mission to educate women and men about the miraculous creative power of the universe contained in the egg and the sperm. When you put into practice what is contained in this book you will discover radiant health and longevity, a calm balanced emotional body. Ultimately, you will release your fear of death, and discover the eternal peace and bliss of your androgynous Soul.

Andrew Kenneth Fretwell,
Founder of www.wuji-gong.org worldwide community

Finally a book for men! Very important information about the man's sexuality, prostate, pelvic floor and more. And I really appreciate the excercises, very useful and effective. Thank's!

Mikael, 35, Data technician

Oh, how I've been looking for a book like this! Many teachings describe the path between the brain and the heart as the longest and most difficult. This book also take you from the root to the heart. A way for the brave!

Stefan, 59, Senior Adviser

CONTENTS

THE MASCULINE ESSENCE

THE PATH OF LIFE

EXERCISES

PREFACE

Ever since "Create Health with Your Sexual Energy: The Tao Approach to Women's Well-Being" – my book about the female sexuality and the feminine essence – came out, I have often gotten the question: When is the book about men's sexual well-being coming out? That idea matured over time and you are now holding the result in your hand: a book about the male sexuality and the masculine essence. It is time to create new representations and stretch our imagination further when it comes to the male sexuality. To get to share these uplifting Taoist Qigong-exercises to men have made this endeavor all the more inspiring and satisfying.

It has been exceedingly fascinating to immerse myself in the writing of this book. The principles in Tao are the same for men and women, but since we look different out of a physiological perspective, the training somewhat varies. We think we know quite a lot about what is male and female and how we function, but there is so much that we don't know about each other. I really recommend all women to read this book as well, and for all men to read the book about women's sexual well-being. They also compliment each other, as I haven't wanted to repeat myself too much when it comes to the sexual Qigong theories and different principles. There are many different ways to illuminate the same subject, and new learnings emerge along the way.

The Taoist exercises are rewarding tools which I have been fascinated by for a long time. Since the middle of the 1990s I have been using these exercises to explore and nurture myself. My own exploration constantly elevates my curiosity and strengthens my will to continue to grow as a person and boost my will to share the teachings. Through the years I have guided and educated many women and men, and I never cease to be amazed by the power these exercises hold. My respect for, and faith in, the ability of the body and mind to heal themselves has intensified and I see it as my mission to help make it possible for that power to take place.

The exercises presented here are primarily inspired by different Taoist teachings and by many of my Qigong teachers; Andrew Fretwell, Wang Ting Jun, David Verdesi, Mantak Chia and Yuan Tze. Other sources of inspiration for this book are what I've learnt from my work as a body therapist and coach, my experience of yoga, Tantra, shamanic body dearmoring and Quodoushka, along with my time at different centers in India. I mix the Taoist theory and modern research about the male anatomy and erotic potential with mine and other people's experiences and studies in alternative therapies, as well as conventionally taught medicine.

Furthermore, I have interviewed and conversed with men about their experiences and practice regarding health, sexuality and about being a man today. I have also been trying to figure out what men would like to read in a book about male sexuality. To enrich the book further I have been interviewing some of my male teachers and colleagues.

The intention of this book is not to create a new macho man, who is able to have endless amounts of sex and who is always ready to go. The intention is neither to create a softy who is only empathetic and meditative. In the new times it is not about being either or, but one and the other. Tao wishes to teach a practical way for both men and women to use their life energy and simultaneously deepen their experience of love and freedom of the soul. There is actually only one way; the one that leads to a deeper connection to yourself and an acceptance of who you are. Regardless of your sexual orientation, if you are romantically inclined or have a spiritual discipline, you can appreciate this knowledge and these practices.

Iréne Andersson, Stockholm, 2020

INTRODUCTION

"Create Health with Your Sexual Energy" gives you access to a reliable source of inner power, confidence and self-reflection. A space within is created, through the exercises, where you can lay the foundation for better health and greater awareness about yourself, your body and your life energy. You get to know your essence, your sexuality and how to elevate your potency and ability for sexual pleasure.

One of the teachings within Taoism is that we all have an incredible inherent potential of possibilities that you can unfold, and which helps us to grow and mature. You, just like a car, need maintenance, lubrication and fuel to function extensively and effectively. Then you won't have to do repairs and exchange as many parts. This book contains knowledge and exercises that will help you find this care and your path to a sustainable life. You get to learn how to be more receptive and responsive to your needs, without losing the connection to your own power. By cultivating your sexual energy you create an intimacy with yourself and trust in your intuition and your senses. For men, this process means that you, among other things, learn how to separate the orgasm from the ejaculation and become multi-orgasmic. Through the exercises in this book you train yourself to individually cultivate your sexual capacity and your awareness of yourself as a human being and as a man. A pleasant side effect is also an elevated vitality and health.

> *Create Health with Your Sexual Energy contains knowledge and exercises that will provide you with tools to cultivate your inherent potential.*

From theory to exercises

The book begins with a theory section on Taoism, Qigong, sexual Qigong and what is meant by "sexual energy". Equally important as learning how to execute a certain technique, is to understand why and the teachings behind it. Following that is a walk-through of the male anatomy and it's erotic potential, regarded in Tao as the foundation to explore the male essence. Taoism also calls attention to the body as the instrument you have at your disposal to explore and develop yourself. The more knowledge and understanding you have about how you function, the better. The last chapter, in regards to theory, deals with the life cycles, prostate awareness and andropause. And last come the exercises specifically designed for men.

The spine and directions for movement

To better understand the text's description of the location of different organs and points, we will go through the spine and directions for movement.

The spine consists of 33 vertebrae, top to bottom:

- 7 neck vertebrae counted from the skull base. They are called cervical vertebrae and termed C1-C7.

- 12 chest vertebrae, each with connected ribs. They are called thoracic vertebrae and termed T1-T12.

- 5 vertebrae in the lower back. They are called lumbar vertebrae and termed L1-L5.

- 5 vertebrae, grown together into the sacrum.

- 4 vertebrae, grown together into the tailbone.

- At the front of the pelvis is the pubic bone.

All movements in the exercises are described in the same way, no matter if you are standing, sitting or laying down.

- Forward intends toward the stomach.

- Backward intends toward the back.

- Down intends toward the feet.

- Up intends toward the head.

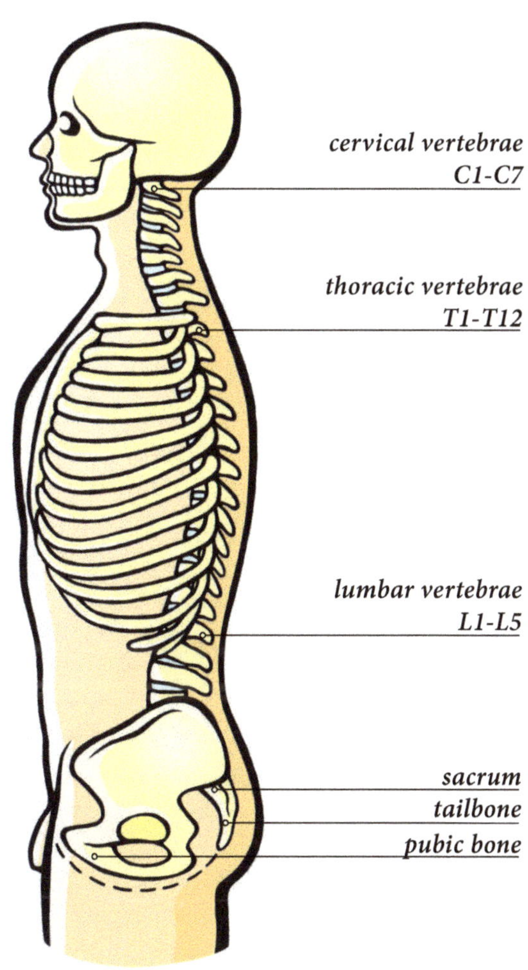

cervical vertebrae
C1-C7
thoracic vertebrae
T1-T12
lumbar vertebrae
L1-L5
sacrum
tailbone
pubic bone

TAOISM
AND SEXUAL QIGONG

Taoism

Tao means "the path" and Taoism presents a philosophy which talks about a natural living in tune with life, nature and a universe of constant change. The Taoists were scientists and free thinkers who developed Taoism thousands of years ago in China. Lao Tzu and Huang Di "The Yellow Emperor" are considered the founders, and their works Dao De Jing "The Classic of Way and Virtue" and Huang Di Nei Jing "The Yellow Emperor's Classic of Internal Medicine" are viewed as the foundational pillars. These works can be hard to interpret and because of that they have cleared the path to many different schools of thought within Tao, even though the foundational principles remain the same. They patiently studied nature, the universe and learned about life. Through practicing this wisdom and applying the principles, the Taoist way arose and different main terminologies and methods for a balanced life were created. According to Tao, you live your life through observing and following the laws of the universe and nature and respecting our planet. Taoism has a holistic worldview where all the things in the universe are connected.

Tao, a path in change

An even older classical work is I Ching, "Book of Changes". The foundational principle is that everything in the universe is in constant change. In the West it's sometimes known as a book that can predict the future. In China it is still diligently used today as a guide to life. It presents images, called trigrams, in change, but as it's a transformation that heed to natural laws it is therefore predictable. Tao suggests that if a development is possible to predict we can adapt and meet the change in a more intelligent way. This attitude makes us the co-creator instead of a victim. You can align yourself with the flow of change and be ready to face and affect your life through true knowledge and wisdom.

An image for this constant dance and striving for balance is the symbol for yin and yang. From the two expressions that are yin and yang derived the five elements, that later became the 64 hexagrams in I Ching (see image on p. 18), which represent the different stages of development. Energy is transformed through different phases and when they are integrated new life emerges. The exercises in this book help you to bring harmony to the transformation and receive life in a more accepting and balanced way.

Energy = matter

Everything is in constant change and transformed from energy to matter and from matter to energy. This is universal law, known from multiple schools of thought and is a conclusion that modern physics also made, for example through Einstein's famous equation E=mc2, energy = mass (speed of light squared), formulated in 1905. We probably haven't fully understood the meaning of this yet since it takes a long time for new thought patterns to permeate our consciousness, as we are often fully occupied with focusing on the material part of ourselves. But the fact of the matter is that if you look at yourself through a microscope you consist of 100 billion cells. These then consist of 20 billion atoms, and when the scientists look even deeper, all they see is energy. The atom core is positively charged and the circulating electrons are negatively charged. Between them are photons, a light phenomena without mass. We are complex energy beings, built from the same small components as the rest of the universe, atoms and even smaller parts. Everything is vibrations, electromagnetism (positive poles and negative poles), which we can perceive or sense intuitively. In quantum mechanics today they are theorizing about Higgs particles in the Higgs field, small components that permeate the entire universe. These force fields are what give other particles mass. The media tend to refer to the Higgs particle as the "God particle".

> *We are all a part of the whole and the collective human soul, in constant transformation and striving towards balance.*

In Taoism, they have studied who we are as human beings and tried to understand the universe through exploring our inner world, which includes both the physical body and the energy body. We all have a physical body and an energy body. They are two parts of the same whole. Where one is visible and the other is invisible. All physical matter is built out of atoms and between these is a "void" with invisible energy. There is a part of our reality that we can't see, but it's still real since we can both affect it and be affected by it. Many older traditions say that the "visible" reality is a mirror image of the "invisible", and that it is in the "invisible" world where the "visible" one is created. According to quantum theory, particles and their counterparts are created constantly.

Yin and yang, the five elements and the eight trigrams.

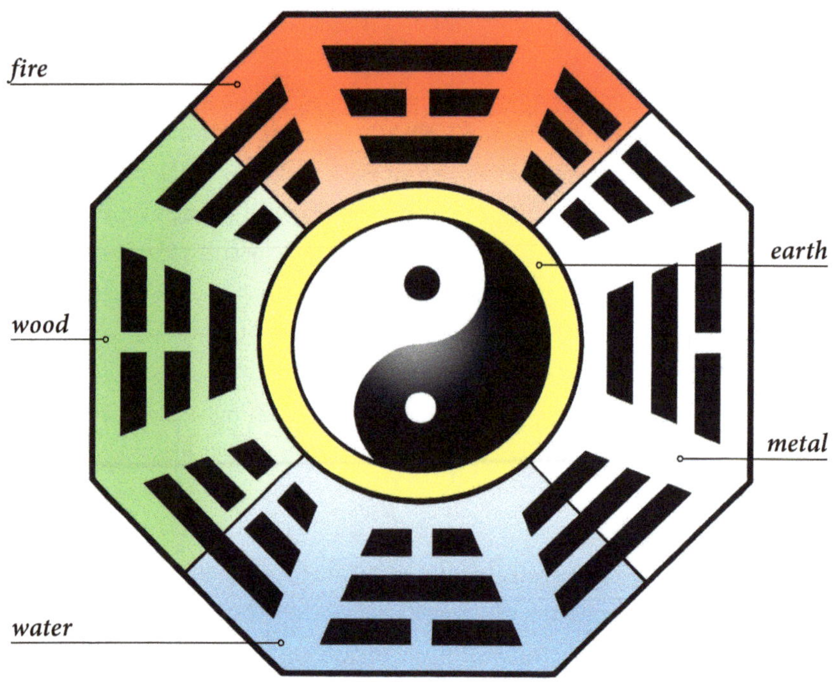

The ancient forces of yin and yang were created out of the void. Followed by the five elements and the eight trigrams. All represent the different qualities and aspects of the universal forces. Different variations of the trigrams create the hexagrams consisting of the 64 transformation variables in "I Ching".
The split line is yin and the complete line is yang.

So the universe is not an empty space between planets or atoms, but a dynamic whole where everything is connected. We are all a part of the whole and the collective human soul, in constant transformation and striving towards balance. Our personal experience as separate beings is merely an illusion.

Another way to describe these correlative parts (energy and materia, positive and negative) is the saying "on earth as it is in heaven" as in the Lord's prayer. Others may speak of as above and so below while Tao speaks about yin and yang.

Yin and Yang

Yin and yang are two well known terms from the Taoist philosophy. They are two opposite forces sprung out of Tao and represent different aspects of the whole. These forces are in constant change, striving for balance and unable to exist without each other. All can be explained by yin and yang and all is relative. Examples of yin and yang are dark and light, cold and warm, night and day, female and male, negative and positive, and so on. An example of their relativity would be that a small light is yang in relation to darkness, but yin in relation to strong sunlight. Between these opposites exists an energy current, much like in electromagnetic fields. These fields also exist inside of us, between men and women, and within everything from the smallest atom to all the planets and great galaxies of the universe.

All people have both yin, feminine aspects, and yang, masculine aspects, within. This is reflected in our brain, where the left side is connected to logical and linear thinking, while the right is connected to a more creative and non-linear thinking. To direct and focus on energy stimulates the cognitive and linear side. To experience and feel stimulates the intuitive and non-linear side. The different scenarios in life demands of you to take different roles and positions regardless of your gender. Balance between the two polarities will promote a richer life.

The importance in restoring the balance between the masculine and feminine within can not be emphasized enough.

Male and female

The male and female are examples of two different forces. The male is associated with yang, an active, fertilizing force with qualities of logic, performance and doing, and related to the external and the known. The female is associated with yin, a receptive, creative energy with qualities like magic, intuition and being, and related to the internal and the unknown. To experience harmony within, regardless of gender, you will need a balance between the active and the receptive and between the logical and illogical.

The society we live in also needs more awareness and balance around this duality. In a society where rational thinking and the external is favored, and the magical and inner dimensions are repressed we risk becoming insensitive to the feminine and to the mystical. Examples of this are where soft values like care and respect for nature and life are downgraded, and also to disregard the magical and healing ability of our own body. Instead we favor reason, growth and being effective without awareness of the consequences.

Both men and women need to see the whole picture and have full acceptance regarding all aspects of life. The importance in restoring the balance between the masculine and feminine within can't be emphasized enough. An equilibrium which can be manifested into life and contribute to finishing the collective war between the patriarchy and matriarchy. Both our relationships and the condition of the world are direct mirrors of ourselves. The change starts with you. By building your knowledge of how yin and yang correlate within, you can act with more awareness and understanding about how we all interact. One interpretation of the message in the book "The Toltec Teachings" (Théun Mares) may be that the most important thing a man needs to do to restore balance in the world is to get your balanced masculine power back and reconquer the connection with your emotional life.

Qigong

One of the foundations in Tao is understanding how we economize our life energy. Taoism is the philosophy and principles behind Qigong, which is the collective name of a number of well-practiced Chinese exercises where Qi stands for life energy and Gong for exercise. Qigong changes, strengthens and balances our life energy.

In the West we have created various techniques for the body - we work out and pump iron. There are plenty of methods to exercise our psyche and our brain, we go to therapy sessions or read self-help books. But none of these deals with our energy body. In all Chinese medicine it is considered fundamental for your health and well-being to take care of your life energy and understand how we can preserve and circulate it inside our bodies.

Qigong relies upon thousands of years of Taoist experience and is the yoga of the Taoists. The different Qigong forms has several Chinese names. I teach, for example, Xing Shen Zhuang, Wuji Gong and Tao Yin. What these techniques have in common is that you focus on the internal and aspire toward good posture and a relaxed body. Slow movements, conscious breathing and meditations are part of the exercises. In Tao, you consider thoughts and feelings to affect the practice and life energy, so learning about how your consciousness works is also included. There are also Qigong-methods used to you train yourself to connect with energy out in the universe, and pull it towards you through your consciousness. You cultivate your own inner universe. The cosmic energy is, according to Tao, infinite and neutral and can be programmed to a strengthening, benign and healthy life energy. Today medical Qigong with focus on better health is common, but in the beginning the practice of Qigong was also a spiritual path, which it still is today for many practitioners.

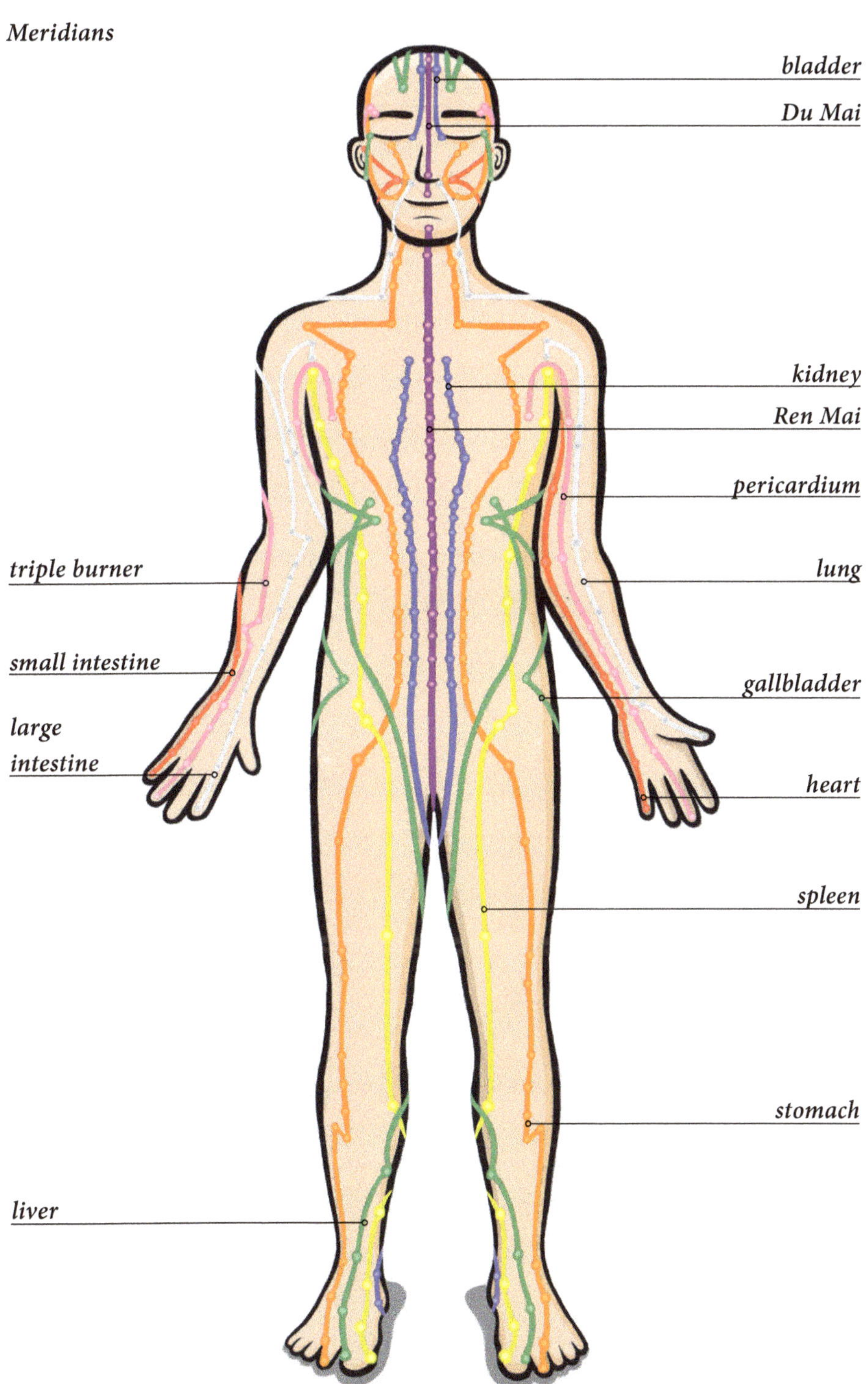

Qi is circulated in the body along energy paths, meridians, which are connected to different organs.

The Qigong practice contributes to better health by strengthening the immune system, giving you greater resilience and lowers your stress levels. The exercises in this book also lead to an increased awareness about your sexual energy as well as the possibility for raised potency and elevated pleasure. For the exercises to have the best effect, it is very important to understand the principles. One who feels encouraged has a lot to receive from these practices which can give surprising revelations and strong experiences.

What is Qi?

Everything has its own specific vibration – its own "vibes" – whether it is a physical manifestation, a feeling, a color, a rock, a person, a cell or an atom. This is something that we are all aware of. Everyone has the ability to read the atmosphere of a room, we directly feel whether a person we meet is happy or sad and we can perceive different impressions from what we see around us. All things have their own Qi, their own energetic pattern. Qi has many different shapes, qualities and intensities and is in constant change. Qi is sometimes explained as electromagnetism. Qi exists within and around us. In this book we will mainly focus on the life energy which exists within. The human body can't exist without Qi; it is the motor itself, according to Tao. Without Qi there is no life. The Taoists talk about good health as in Qi being balanced. When a disease appears it means your Qi is out of balance, weakened or there is an excess of it.

Qi is life energy. According to Tao, good health is about balancing your Qi. When diseases appear it means your Qi is out of balance, weakened or there is an excess of it.

Meridians

Qi circulates within the body along the meridians. On the meridians there are points which are affected during acupuncture treatments. Through reading the pulse of the meridians (fast, slow, weak, strong) and quality (moist, dry, warm, cold) the practitioner of acupuncture can detect imbalances before they can cause too much damage to the body.

There are twelve primary meridians connected to different inner organs, along with eight other channels, out of which we will study three: Du Mai (the meridian going up the spine), Ren Mai (the meridian guided down the front of the body) and Chong Mai (the thrusting channel, through the middle of the body). These are the meridians which are most talked about in Qigong, but there are more. For the energy to flow unhindered through these energy paths, it's important that the body is relaxed and balanced. You may say that Qigong can work as a form of self-acupuncture. It is said that in old China the practitioner of acupuncture only received payment as long as the patient remained healthy, as it was the task of the practitioner to discover imbalances before they manifested as diseases. It is better to prevent the illness than to cure it later.

Besides acupuncture, traditional Chinese medicine consists of herbs, Qigong and massage and by tradition also astrology and Feng Shui. They also use the "five elements theory" to diagnose and describe symptoms and conditions. Fire, earth, metal, water and wood represent the different aspects and characteristics in us and are associated with the inner organs. Tao teaches that all aspects of life can be reflected in the elements. Read more about the elements along with the exercise the inner smile on p. 105.

Qi has three parts

Qi consists of three aspects; matter, energy and information and they all affect each other. You have a body, you have an energy body and you have a consciousness. Your physical body is the matter. Your energy body vibrates your feelings and Qi flowing in the meridians. Information exists in your consciousness in the form of your thoughts, attitudes and approach, and as spiritual connection. Your cells and organs are programmed by your DNA and heritage, and they know which tasks they have been assigned. But your consciousness also affects the cell biology and the surroundings in which they act.

"Energy follows thought" is a well known concept which is important to understand for the exercises in this book. Thought is energy and you affect it's direction. By alternating your focus, you are able to guide the Qi in your body. It is your thoughts in your consciousness which supplies your Qi with information. "It will be as you thought", is what Olof Röhlander (popular swedish lecturer in the power of the mind) usually says, as he asks his audience, "so what did you think?" Are you thinking thoughts which strengthen you and make you feel well? Or are you thinking thoughts that deflate yourself and make you feel worthless? The human being has a tragic ability to seek affirmations in that one is just as worthless as one thinks. It is you who decide what ideas and attitudes you have, and through these you become the co-creator of your own life. In the light of this knowledge, it becomes easier to realize the importance of learning more about how our consciousness works and become increasingly aware of different thought patterns. It is empowering to find an attitude which leads to sustainable change in the desired direction as well as a humility towards what life is offering. You can't affect everything that happens in your life, but you can affect your attitude and how you handle different situations.

But from where is the information coming? Yuan Tze, Qigong teacher, describes it as this: *Most phenomena act out their own 'laws'. An animal or a plant lives according to their programming and instinct. They don't have autonomy. In this respect the information is objective. The human consciousness is more complex and can take its own initiatives and has its own ideas and thoughts. Furthermore, humans are equipped with the ability of development and self-realization. Our consciousness has the potential to be awake and alert all the time. We create and affect our life, our body and life energy through our consciousness. Every thought you have affects yourself and your surroundings. The thoughts send information in which strength and intensity varies. What can your consciousness achieve? It can actually influence space. There is nothing your consciousness can't affect.*

According to Tao it is essential also for humans to keep within our "laws". These laws include qualities such as respect for all life, trust, honesty, love and hopefulness as well as aspiring toward keeping balance and health. Our modern lifestyle tends to break the boundaries of these laws, unfortunately, which makes us contributors in creating unbalance, both internally and externally.

Sex and spirituality

Sexual energy is a foundational force in our universe. Everything that's alive comes from this creational power. Sexual energy has an incredibly strong and magical affect. If we go past the reproduction in itself, it becomes even more remarkable and ineffable. Some would say that this is what separates us from animals, that we can choose to have sex purely out of pleasure. With the help of our consciousness we can also elevate our sexuality to a "higher" level, far away from our everyday selves. The orgasm can open to love and ecstasy, a heightening experience of a deeply human touch and affinity. Gaining unique knowledge beyond time and space. Spiritual experiences or awakenings are often described as something timeless and greater than ourselves. People have always had spiritual experiences and different approaches to spirituality. We can have awakenings in various contexts, through spiritual teachers, meetings, nature, meditation, books, childbirth etc. Our understanding of these experiences are minimal though, especially here in the West. One reason is that they can't be explained scientifically. The way in which people interpret their religion has also contributed to why some look at their spiritual experiences with fear or doubt. It is often in correlation to an orgasm that we experience a heightened or spiritual awareness. Strong spiritual experiences and intense love events often lead to a greater trust in life and a lust to live more fully.

Several older schools of thought talk about sexuality as both holy and healing. They describe how you can embody the spirit, or spiritualize the body, and even fill your entire body and being with orgasmic ecstasy. When all our energy centers within our body, or our chakras, as the Indian teachings call them, are ignited, we have become enlightened and reached full consciousness. In her excellent book about the theology of the body Sister Sofie is interpreting Pope John Paul II: "The human body was created to transfer into the visible reality of the world the mystery hidden since time immemorial in God, and thus be a sign of it". The union between man and woman is an analogy for the mysterious union between the soul and God.

Most spiritual schools have different paths and maps for development and training of the human consciousness toward completion, and all include different ways to handle and regulate sexual energy. From sexual abstinence and joining a monastery, circulating divine energy in Tantra, a philosophy and spiritual practice originating from India, exploring different sides of your personality in the shamanic love art Quodoushka from "the twisted hairs elders", a traditional heritage from the American continents, to various old fertility rituals. Sexuality and spirituality appears to belong together. In the collection of essays "Sex – för guds skull", "Sex – for God's Sake" they even ask the question: "Religion and sex, how can you separate them?" The text revolves around sexuality and erotica in the great world religions and how they have acquainted themselves with what is good and bad sexuality. But our sexuality is a neutral force and spirituality in itself belongs to no specific religion, but is something that is present within all of us.

If you had complete integrity in your sexual drives it would probably be a revolution in your way of creating relationships.

In China, they have long since discovered that the key to a long life of happiness and health is the cultivation of sexual energy. They invented these Taoist exercises and created sexual Qigong to make use of this infinite source of energy. So what is sexual Qigong and what can it give you? We begin by investigating additional terms and some theoretical base knowledge before we start the exercises.

Sexuality and our culture

The information given to us on how we ought to relate to our sexuality, and the social imprinting from our culture, has nothing to do with who, or what we are at our core. It will tell us how we should act and present ourselves and is based on the ideas and values of other people, our society and our religions. This means that what is normative for sexuality, what is right and wrong, and what is masculine or feminine differentiates depending on culture and time periods.

Many fear the power of sexuality, which is evident in several religious practices in the world. Women are forced to hide their bodies so that men won't lose control over their urges and end up in unexpected indignations. Different schools of thought demonstrate various ways of handling sexuality and there are sometimes clearly defined rules of what a "worthy sexuality" looks like. Many people will unfortunately not fit into these parameters and experience great difficulty in their battle to fit in. Suppression of the subconscious is what makes a person's sexuality hard to maneuver. Energy which is pushed down gathers like water in a pond. It takes a lot of energy to keep it suppressed and when it is relegated to the subconscious it will get a life of its own. The sexual energy can then take a different expression as perversions or violence. When you affirm your sexuality as a neutral force you become more balanced. By getting to know yourself, you find security. It's about making these values and attitudes conscious and in turn free yourself of what doesn't serve you. Your lust is neither good nor evil, but proof of your creativity and hunger for life.

Sexual energy

The role that sexual energy plays in the Taoist exercises are probably different from what you're accustomed to think about and relate to the amorous power. This is because sexual energy doesn't have that much to do with sexuality in an ordinary sense. It's not about sexual monogamy regulated to a bedroom, where it in the worst case scenario would be used as an outlet for frustration or an expression of an undetermined longing. Instead it is viewed as a neutral energy, a creative potential with an intelligence that can support your training and your life in all kinds of fantastic ways. Sexual energy is in itself objective and without moral judgements of what is good or bad.

Is it possible to free your sexuality from personal and cultural values? It is common to weigh your sexuality down with guilt and shame. Let it instead, regardless of your own life history, be whatever force it is, without judging it for what you think is right or wrong. Not as an uncontrolled drive, but with integrity and respect for both yourself and others. You can't change your past but you can always change your attitude, and in this way recreate the now in an instant.

Gaining access to and cultivating your sexual energy is the foundation of this practice. A transformation where through individual cultivation you learn how to guide the energy into your body rather than projecting it outward.

Try to imagine how you would choose a partner if your attraction was not governed by more or less unsatisfied erotic cravings and subconscious emotional needs. That does not mean that lust isn't there, but that it's more intentional and closer connected to the real wish and desires of your heart.

> *Gaining access to and cultivating your sexual energy is the foundation of this training. You learn how to guide the energy into your body rather than projecting it outward.*

The libido runs reproduction and our ability to reproduce is a strong biological instinct. Sexual acts naturally strengthen romantic relationships, but it is also linked with our creative power and the creational force of the universe. To refine our awareness of, and connectedness to, this energy, with or without a partner, is a part of the Taoist sexology.

Sexual Qigong

The notion that sexual energy has a both holy and healing potential is something the Taoists have known for thousands of years. The Chinese Tao masters observed that our sexual functions were closely related to physical and psychological health. They also saw that it was the foundation for both personal development and for where to cultivate spiritual capacities. This involves intentional engagement with the sexual energy. A path for this cultivation of sexual energy is to be celibate. Celibacy restrains us from sexual relations and sexual activity, to focus on conserving our life force and spiritual development instead. The purpose of the sexual Qigong practice is then to stop having sex and rid oneself of the need derived from lust. But there is also another way, and that is to learn how to cultivate the life force energy while living an ordinary and sexually active life. Sexual Qigong involves intentional engagement with the sexual energy.

Sexual alchemy

The feminine and masculine is described as a negative pole and a positive pole. We also have different charges in different places of our bodies. A man is positively (yang) charged in the genitals and negatively (yin) charged in the heart, while for the woman it is reversed. This means that a woman gives from her heart and receives in her genitals and the man gives with his genitals and his sexuality and receives in the heart. Men help women to open up sexually and women help men to open up their heart. An immature expression is that a woman "just wants to get married" and a man "just wants to have sex" without respect for the partner. We often misinterpret each other, overthinking these signals and react unconsciously and with judgement. Men may perceive women as demanding when they look for emotional confirmation and women may perceive men to be threatening when they express their sexual desires. It is not rare that the reactions are that both withdraw instead of affirming the energies to explore the actual situation and what the other is implying. How can we respect and handle these differences in our foundational energy? Through contact with both your emotional life and your sexuality there will be no unconscious charge regarding sex or emotions that needs to be avoided. Strive to affirm both your own longings and the longings of others and consider them reasonable and natural. To be honest and not repressing your libido or emotions creates self-esteem and integrity.

The man's genitals and the woman's heart being the positive pole also means that the

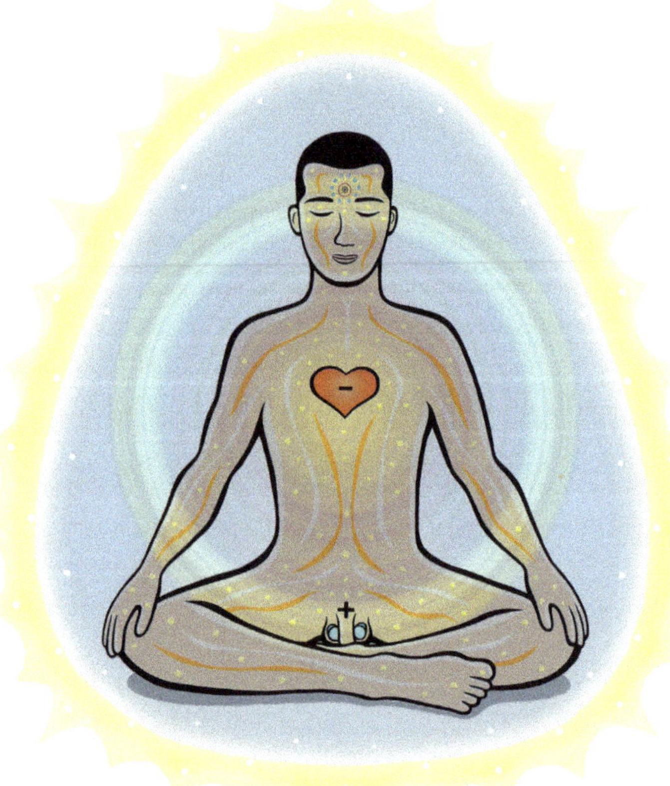

All is energy. All is electromagnetic fields with positive and negative charges. The man has his positive pole in his genitals and his negative pole in his heart. For the woman it is the other way around.

sexual arousal of women starts in the heart and goes toward the genitals, that is from love to sex, and for men it is the other way around, from sex to love. The sensation in the male's genitals arouses interest and hopefully becomes the path to lovingness and opening of the heart. As this connection between your genitals and heart strengthens, your body will wake up to both sexuality and love.

Sexual Qigong in theory

All of us are born with a certain potential for vitality, characterized by the conception and union between our parents and what we inherit from them. This combination gives us a certain amount of basic life energy. This innate energy is called Jing and stands for human essence, sperm generative energy, drive and longing to reproduce. Jing also fuels our sexuality, hormone production and creativity. Our heritage is complemented by the energy we receive from the food we eat and the air we breathe. Even when we spend time in nature, rest or exercise we gain new power.

You also use energy in, for example, work, digestion and various activities. As the years pass, depending on your lifestyle, you start overdrawing your energy resources and increasingly take more and more from the reserves. Your vital organs, glands, and finally the brain, become overloaded. You start consuming more than you add, and your aging accelerates. According to the Taoists, it is a very energy-intensive process for the body to produce eggs and sperm. The woman predominately loses vitality through heavy menstruations and the man through the production and ejaculation of sperm. Therefore, some of the exercises in this book are designed to reduce these processes, and they differ slightly for men and women.

A money pouch

A single ejaculation contains many million sperms, each of which has the potential to create life. The tail of each little sperm vibrates with 40 strokes per second and would they all be able to reach and fertilize one egg each, you could become the father of Europe's entire population. According to the Taoists, sperm is man's most essential Qi and when you lose your sperm, you lose that power. So of course, this depletes your life energy. The sperms are formed in the testicles and their value is so great that we can easily confirm that you are wearing a real "money pouch". Therefore, according to Tao, men feel best if they do not always ejaculate in sexual activity.

At the same time you have an abundance of innate sexual energy, which is a power which seems infinite and it's also the only force that can be multiplied. For many of us, merely a thought is literally enough to speed up our orgasmic flow. It is this Jing force that you use, recycle and refine in sexual Qigong. Raw sexual energy becomes nutrition for body and soul.

The three treasures of life energy

For a deeper understanding of the transformational potential of Taoism, we need to clarify the concept of "the three treasures of life energy" (San Bao in Chinese). They are described in terms of Jing (sexual energy), Qi (life energy) and Shen (spiritual energy). Generally speaking, and very simplified, the purpose of the training can be described as transforming sexual energy into life energy and, in turn, to spiritual energy or expansion of your counsciousness. This act is called "the three treasures of life energy". They are all different aspects of the same thing. This transformation takes place in different parts of the body and by guiding and circulating energy. Three important places are the three Dan Tian, elixir fields or energy centers for storing Qi. If the meridians are like rivers in the body where energy can flow, these are lakes where energy can be gathered. Lower Dan Tian is an area of the lower abdomen, behind and below the navel and will be the most important area for these exercises. There is also middle Dan Tian, behind the sternum, in the heart center and upper Dan Tian behind the third eye, in the middle of the forehead, and into the head.

> *Jing, sexual energy, is a force which seems infinite, and it is also the force that can be multiplied.*

You can learn how to convert your sexual power as well as energy from food, air and your environment, to Qi, which supplies your bodily organs with the necessary energy. This in turn is transformed into Shen - consciousness or spiritual energy. In Qigong, our life force is described based on these three concepts - Jing, Qi and Shen.

Jing = our original energy, our essence, sperm generative energy, sexual power, hormones and reproductive capacity. Linked to our heritage and DNA. Associated with the physical body and the kidneys. The kidneys is described as the batteries of your body, and the carrier of the original Yin and Yang. This is where our fuel is.

Qi = life force, life energy, vitality. Associated with the energy body and all kinds of movement, emotions, breathing, circulation and the flow of the meridians. If Jing is the fuel in the batteries then this is the electricity.

Shen = spiritual energy, consciousness, the soul reflected in the eyes. Associated with the heart, wisdom, compassion and enlightenment. This is the light which radiates

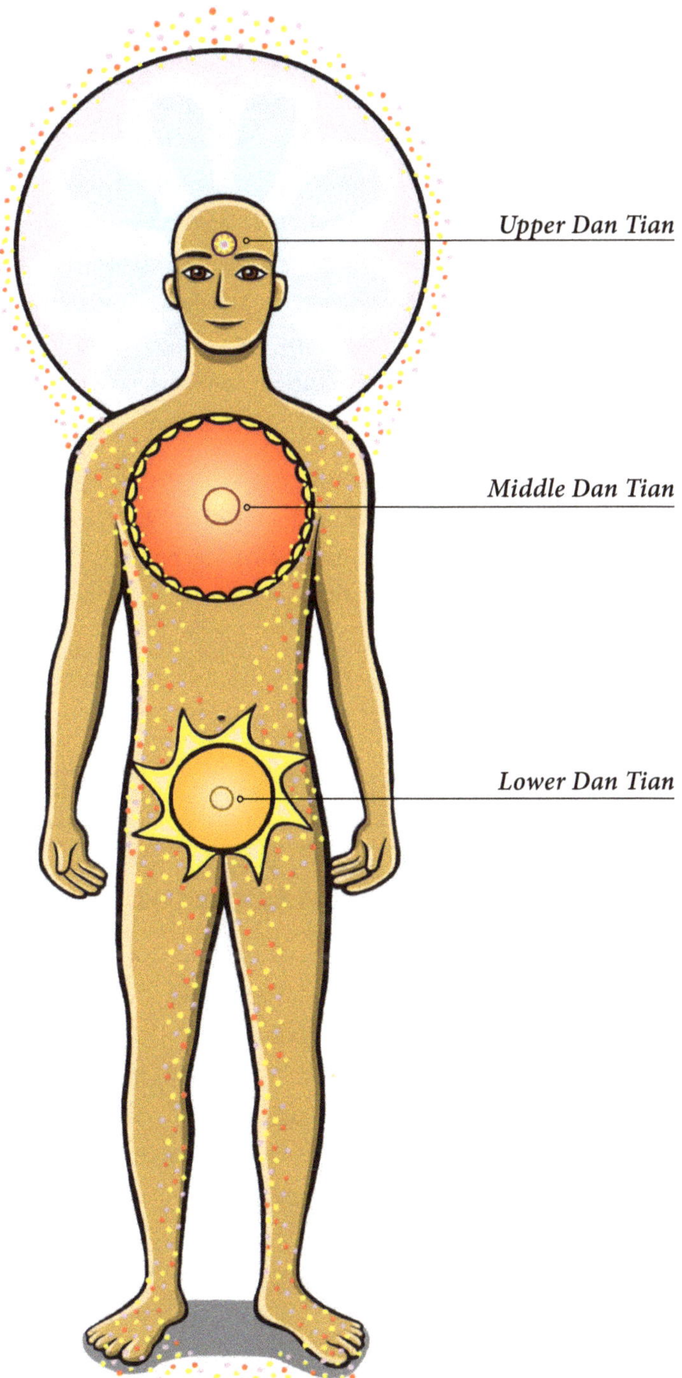

Jing, Qi and Shen are transformed by guiding and circulating energy in different parts of your body. Three important places are the three Dan Tian. In this context the Lower Dan Tian will be of most importance.

from the electricity.

One can also say that the three treasures of life energy vibrate at different frequencies. Jing is the most dense and the slowest and vibrates at a "lower" level, while Shen is more subtle and the fastest and vibrates at a "higher" level. The human mind has the ability to tune in to the different frequencies, just like setting a radio to different wavelengths. Everything changes with the direction, feeling and attitude of your consciousness. It is easier to make changes in our energy bodies and in our consciousness, but not always simple. Everyone knows how difficult it is to change a mindset. Jing, Qi and Shen interact and affect each other. In western conventional medicine, one can only take into account the physical, Jing, which can be seen and touched. On the other hand, it is difficult to measure the other two levels, Qi and Shen, which is a scientific limitation.

Tao works towards a healthy and conscious balance between the three treasures of life energy. It is in the magical intersection between Shen (consciousness), Qi (breathing) and Jing (body) where healing and growth can happen. That is where all becomes one in true serenity and presence.

Lower Dan Tian

Lower Dan Tian, the area of the lower abdomen, behind and below the navel, is an important place in all the exercises. It's a gathering place where energy can be stored to "charge your life energy", depositing it into your "energy account". Energy can be generated and stored safely here and your body can easily absorb it. The more robust and active this center is, the more physically and sexually strong a man will be.

Your original energy, Jing, moves from your kidneys and down to your genitals, where it transforms into sexual secretion and hormones. The sexual organs are best at creating energy, the internal organs of the lower torso are good at collecting energy and the brain is best at receiving and projecting energy. By means of the exercises, sexual energy is transformed and refined through the small circulation (see exercise p. 112). As you learn to circulate the energy through your body, along the spine and into the meridian system, your whole body is vitalized. Regular focus in the lower Dan Tian supports this process. By regularly breathing down into Dan Tian, you strengthen your life energy and create the conditions for Jing, Qi and Shen to be transformed and balanced. Developing the capacities of the lower Dan Tian will increase your sense of grounding and feeling of trust, safety and stability in life. This will also affect your physical and psychological health a lot. Ming Men, in the lower back, is an important point for this process and means the "Gate of Life" (see p. 113).

Your observational skill

Dan Tian is also a neutral place where you can base your experiences and grow your observational ability. The function is there from the outset, but you need to provide the area with attention and your presence for its potential to be fulfilled. It is also from here you can filter your experiences and increase your ability to perceive a phenomena which appears in your consciousness. You become aware that you have a consciousness, another focus point within yourself, which can observe yourself from a distance. Conscious awareness is the key to both increased responsiveness and prolonged enjoyment. It is the foundation for quality in your development. You exercise the consciousness to stay grounded in the body and you become more present.

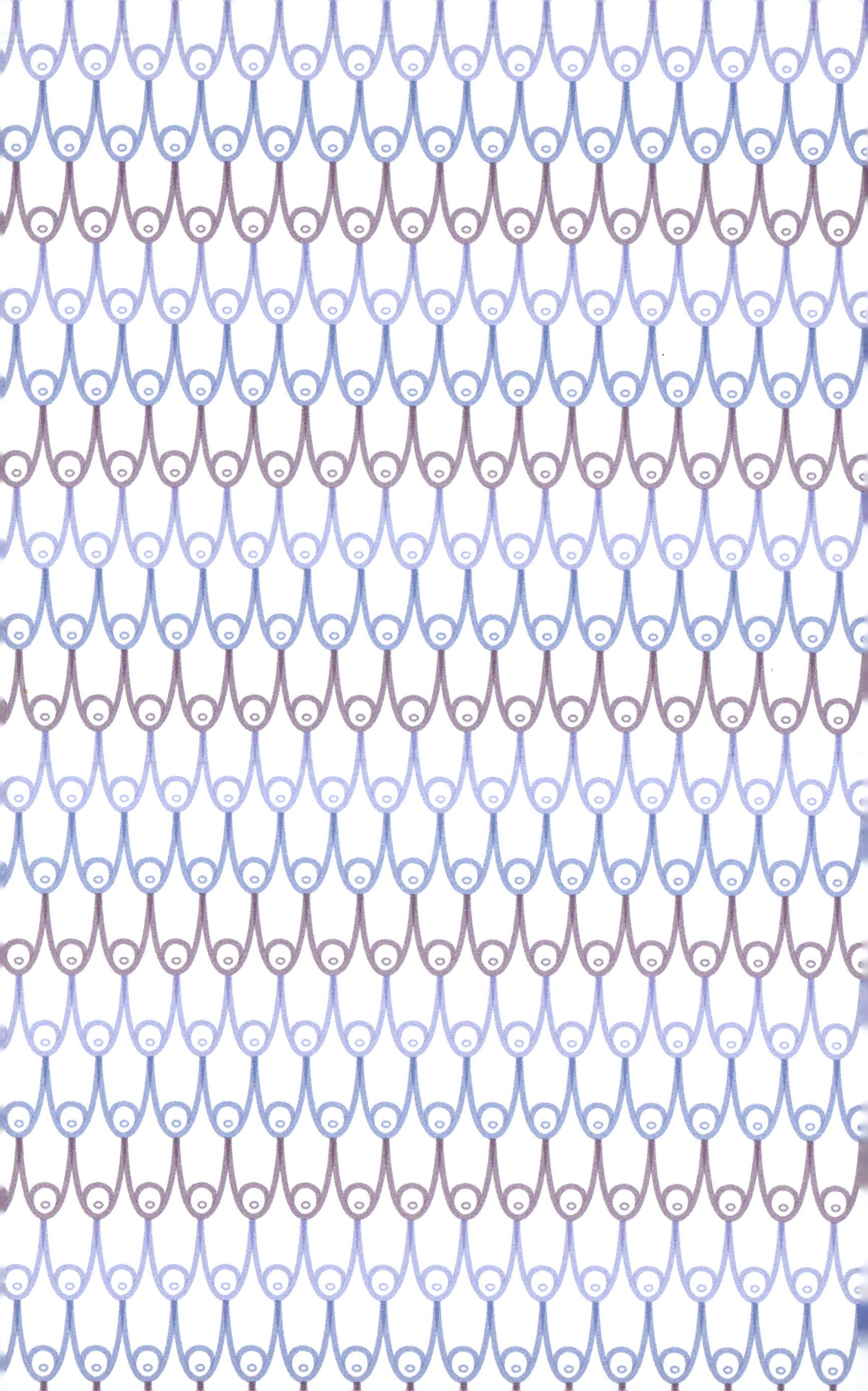

MALE
ANATOMY

The male genitalia and sexual function have been mapped out for a long time. The attributes are easily visible and have a clear task and direction. Since the male body has to work in order to make children a reality, it has always been important for the limb to function properly. The anatomy of the female genitalia on the other hand, wasn't scientifically explored until the 1990s. The woman becomes pregnant, whether she knows how her genitals look or how she works sexually, and whether she enjoys intercourse, or not. At the same time, her sexual capacity has been well rewritten in recent decades and her multi-orgasmic ability has been accepted. It is gratifying to hear how many people have become multi-orgasmic since they have been told that it is possible. The number of multi-orgasms has tripled and studies show that more than half of all women experience multi-orgasms.

The same should also apply to men. As you learn more about your orgasmic capacity, you can get your body and mind to understand what is actually possible. Even men want to refine their erotic nature and have a need to increase and intensify their pleasure. It's high time to put the myth that men are only interested in quick release on the shelf. Knowledge brings new ideas, and practice gives skills, and suddenly it's happening - you've acquired the ability for extended enjoyment as well as multi-orgasms.

Below you'll find information about the anatomy of male genitalia and sexuality, for you to deepen your understanding of how things function in the body. Tao emphasizes the importance of learning as much as possible about your own body, the instrument you have at your disposal for your personal and spiritual development and where you will live for the rest of your life.

Male genital anatomy

The male genitals consists of penis, scrotum, testicles, prostate, seminal vesicles, vas deferens, cowpers glands, urethra, bladder, erectile tissue, muscles, blood vessels and nerves. The variations in size and appearance of the genitals vary greatly among men. The size, form, colour, amount of semen, its taste and the number of times it sprays during ejaculations are different. The differences are also related to variations in the psyche and what stimulation works best. This is well documented knowledge in, for example, Tao and Quodoushka, where differences in male anatomy are a whole theory of different body types with different ways of responding and being excited. Men appreciate pressure, touch and positions in different ways. They get turned on from different things and can be seduced in different ways. Everyone has different temperaments, sensitivity and preferences. We are all unique in our expression and appearance yet continually the same. Full acceptance of your genital sense of self is part of your journey and healing.

Penis

The penis has erectile tissue which fills with blood and becomes hard during sexual arousal, leading to erection. The penis has three parts, cura penis, bulbus penis and glans penis. Cura penis is what we call the spongy structure found on the sides of the penis shaft. At the center is the bulbus penis, the spongy-like tissue surrounding the urethra. The tissue continues into the body a bit and is embedded in muscles, which can be felt through the perineum. The glans penis is the outermost part of the penis which is covered completely or partially by the foreskin. The area on the bottom of the

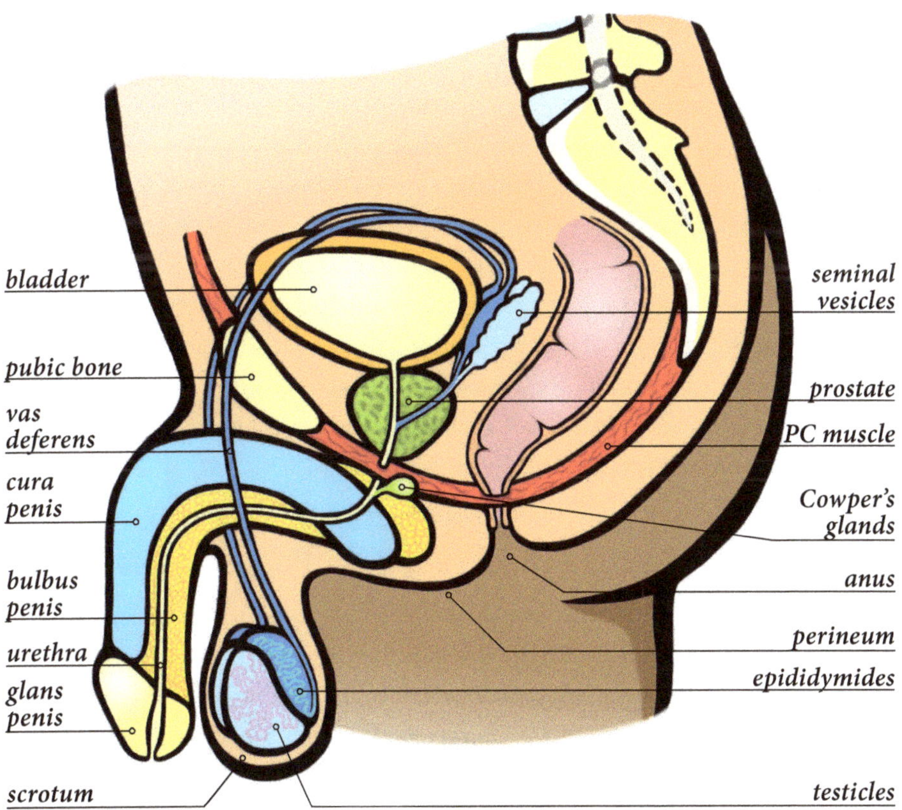

glans penis, where the foreskin attaches, is called the frenulum, and is a very sensitive area for touch. Neither the size or shape of the penis is important for how much pleasurable sex you can have, either for yourself or for the other.

Urethra

The urethra goes from the bladder, via the prostate, through the bulbus penis and is the outbound channel for both urine and ejaculation. When a man has an erection, the opening closes to the bladder. The edges around the mouth of the urethra are often very sensitive to touch, but may require a lot of moisture or lubricants to make it feel comfortable.

Bladder

The bladder is located above the prostate. The urine is stored here before it is excreted through the urethra. The walls of the urinary bladder and prostate are made of muscular layers which allow for urination.

Scrotum

The scrotum is a pouch-like structure hanging below the penis. It contains the testicles.

Testicles

The scrotum holds the testicles, two egg-shaped gonads, around 0,7x1x1,5 inch large, which produce semen and male sex hormones. Each testicle consists of several hundred thin tubes which together are more than 500 yards long. Sperm production takes place in the tubes, and between them are the cells that produce the androgens, the most important being testosterone. The reason for the location of the testicles is that the process of forming works best at about 95-96.8 °F which is lower than normal body temperature which is 98.6 °F.

Epididymis

The epididymis consists of an approximately 0,24 inch wide, twisted and spun, 5 yard long tube on the outside of the testicle where the sperms mature and are stored. It takes two weeks for a sperm to mature in the epididymis, and after three weeks of storage the sperms are released via ejaculation. If ejaculation fails, they break down and the body's cleaning system takes them away.

Sperm

The male reproductive cells are called sperm. The word sperm comes from Greek and means seed. The sperm fertilizes the woman's egg. In total, it takes 2-3 months for a sperm to develop into fertile sperm. A man usually forms about 100 million sperms per day and there are as many as 10 to 200 million per ml (5 ml = 1 teaspoon) in an ejaculation. The sperm count is affected by the number of ejaculations and the time between the ejaculations. Sperm is formed all the time and during the period of a man's most fertile age, the number of sperms is said to be optimal again within a week. The renewal period increases with age. Unfortunately, it seems that our modern lifestyle has affected the number and quality of sperm count negatively (see more p. 86). The right temperature is also important, if it is too hot the sperm production will stop. There are reports from occupations, such as bakers, who have shown reduced sperm production. Even tight underwear are devastating as they push the scrotum towards the body where it gets too hot. The testicles are best placed to hang where they are going, below the body.

Cowper's glands

Cowper's glands are two to the count and about 0,3 inch in size. They are located below the prostate. The glands are intercalated in the pelvic floor muscles on each side of the bulbus penis. Cowper's glands is responsible for producing a pre-ejaculate fluid, a transparent liquid, that comes out of the penis and moisturises the glans. The fluid prepares and cleans the urethra for the sperm. The first drops come early during the erection, so the fluid also acts as a lubricant during intercourse. It also helps create a favorable environment in the vagina for the sperm, and should not contain sperm, but can, so be aware. The female counterpart is called Bartholin's glands.

Semen

The semen consists of three parts; sperm (10-20%), secretion from the seminal vesicles (60%) and secretion from the prostate gland (20-30%). The average amount of semen per ejaculation is approximately 0,1-10 ml. The amount of sprays varies and the same goes for the intensity. It has been shown that the nutritional value of semen is very large, besides sperm, the fluid contains proteins, enzymes, vitamins, minerals and amino acids. The texture and appearance of the fluid can vary, but are usually white, gray or yellowish, thick and sticky, not clear and thin. The taste varies, from salt to bitter, and is influenced by what you eat and by the biochemistry in your body. Unpleasant taste and odor or discolored ejaculate indicates unbalance. If it is red, pink or brown red, it may be because it contains blood. Most often, a small vessel has broken from strain, which is quite common. If the semen is discolored often, consult a physician to investigate the cause, it can for example be an infection.

According to Tao, all your erotic flows is part of your essence.

Vas deferens

Vas deferens (ductus deferens) are tubes that transport sperm fluid from the testicles through the prostate to the urethra. They are about half a yard long.

Prostate

The prostate is a walnut-sized gland that consists of a network of elastic muscles, fibers and blood vessels. It contains a collection of thirty to forty saclike glands. It is also known as the Skene's glands and ducts. The glands secrete through the ejaculatory ducts at the time of ejaculation. The secretion is thin and milky and contributes about one third of the semen and gives it its white color. However, the color may vary slightly between men and on different occasions.

The prostate eliminates PSA (prostate specific antigen), an enzyme whose task is to make it easier for the sperm to swim. The secrete is mildly bascic which helps to neutralize the acidic environment in the vagina, which prolongs the life of the sperm. In addition, the gland produces a small amount of fluid that protects the testicles and urethra from infections. The word prostate means "protector" or "guardian". To function properly it needs androgens, the male sex hormones.

When the penis is stimulated, the prostate swells up with secretion fluids. The vas deferens pass through the prostate before they enter the urethra and seminal fluids gather here before ejaculation. The smooth muscle of the prostate helps to squeeze the sperms out upon release. The prostate is sometimes called the P-zone of men and orgasm can be achieved through stimulation. The prostate is an erotic body (read more p. 62).

Seminal vesicles

The seminal vesicles are two glands about 1,5 inches long, situated behind and above the prostate and between the bladder and rectum. The vesicles exude a secretion that consists of proteins that coagulate after release. The fluid also contains fructose that supports sperm with energy and nutrition. The seminal vesicles empty their fluid after the sperm and prostate secretion and contributes about two thirds of the semen. It is currently unclear what function all of the seminal vesicles secretion has. One guess is that part of its fluid is unfavorable to the vitality of the sperm and blocks up after the sperms, so that no one else's sperm can reach the egg inside the vagina.

Ejaculation

Upon release, the sperms are collected from the epididymis. The sperms move through the vas deferens into the prostate, where they are mixed with secretions from the glands in the prostate just before ejaculation. Lastly the seminal vesicles release their fluid. Thereafter, muscle activity begins to squeeze all ejaculation fluid through the urethra. Then the prostate recovers. Each time the prostate contracts and then becomes relaxed, it draws the ejaculate from glands and vesicles. Then the prostate muscles tighten and push out the fluid through the urethra. The number of sprays and amounts of ejaculate varies between men and depend on their anatomy. A strong healthy man may have powerful contractions during the ejaculation, while a man with prostate problems may only have a few and significantly weaker. Since muscle contractions, both in the prostate and pelvic floor affect ejaculation, untrained pelvic floor muscles may affect the release.

Perineum

Perineum is the area between the anus and the scrotum. There are a lot of nerve endings that make the area sensitive. In this area you can find the "million dollar spot" that can prevent ejaculation by pressure (see p. 137). Touch behind scrotum, towards anus, with light fingers, until you reach a pit, slightly before the anus. This is also an important acupuncture point called Hui Yin. The area is sometimes referred to as the P-zone.

P-zone

The P-zone is an erotic zone that is linked to the prostate. It can be stimulated via the perineum or anus. Via the anus you will find the prostate approximately 2 inches in the front rectum wall. The prostate becomes more sensitive during strong excitement, and stimulation can give a different type of orgasm than that which penis stimulation provides. The P-zone is associated with the female G-zone, and the erectile tissue where the G-zone is located is more frequently being called "the female prostate". In both men and women, science has confirmed huge amounts of sensitive nerve endings around the prostate.

By accident, docent Olle Johansson, at the Karolinska Institute, "found" the man's P-zone when he researched how the human body is affected by microwaves in our environment. In this case, it was about the increase in prostate cancer and he looked at tissue samples from the prostate area in both healthy and ill men. He surprisingly saw the huge concentration of nerve threads surrounding the prostate. It indicates that the nerves are important for a sexual function.

Pelvic floor muscles

The pelvic floor muscles consist of the pelvic diaphragm, muscles which line up as a hammock between the pubic bone and the tailbone. The most important is the PC muscle which is placed closest to the prostate and anus. Below that is the urogenital diaphragm, a group of transverse muscles in the front part of the pelvic floor. At the bottom there are sphincter muscles around the penis root and anus. All of these muscles are essential to your sexual health and to stimulate or prevent ejaculation. Read more about your pelvic floor muscles and exercises on page 130.

Anus

An erogenous zone for many men as the anus is placed close to the prostate. There are also a lot of nerve endings in this area.

Nipples

Several men are surprised by how sensitive their nipples actually can be. They are an erogenous zone for men as well, even though it can take time to awaken the sensitivity.

Nerves and brain

There are several nerves associated with the orgasm. The pudendal nerve is an important orgasm nerve for both men and women. For men it's connected to the penis and the scrotum. The pelvic nerves are a complex of nerves which are important for the erection and are linked to the erectile tissue of the penis, prostate and seminal vesicles. The hypogastric nerve is connected to the testicles and prostate and contributes to the emission. Even the vagus nerve is very important and involved in man's pleasure. It has long been known within Tao and Tantra that the vagus nerve is activated via relaxation and meditation, and it is important both for sensory perceptions as well as for feeling. It constitutes a major part of the parasympathetic nervous system and is therefore essential both for recovery and reversal of the erotic flow. It also affects the throat and palate. The pudendal nerve and pelvic nerve converge further up with the hypoglossal nerve, which controls the tongue.

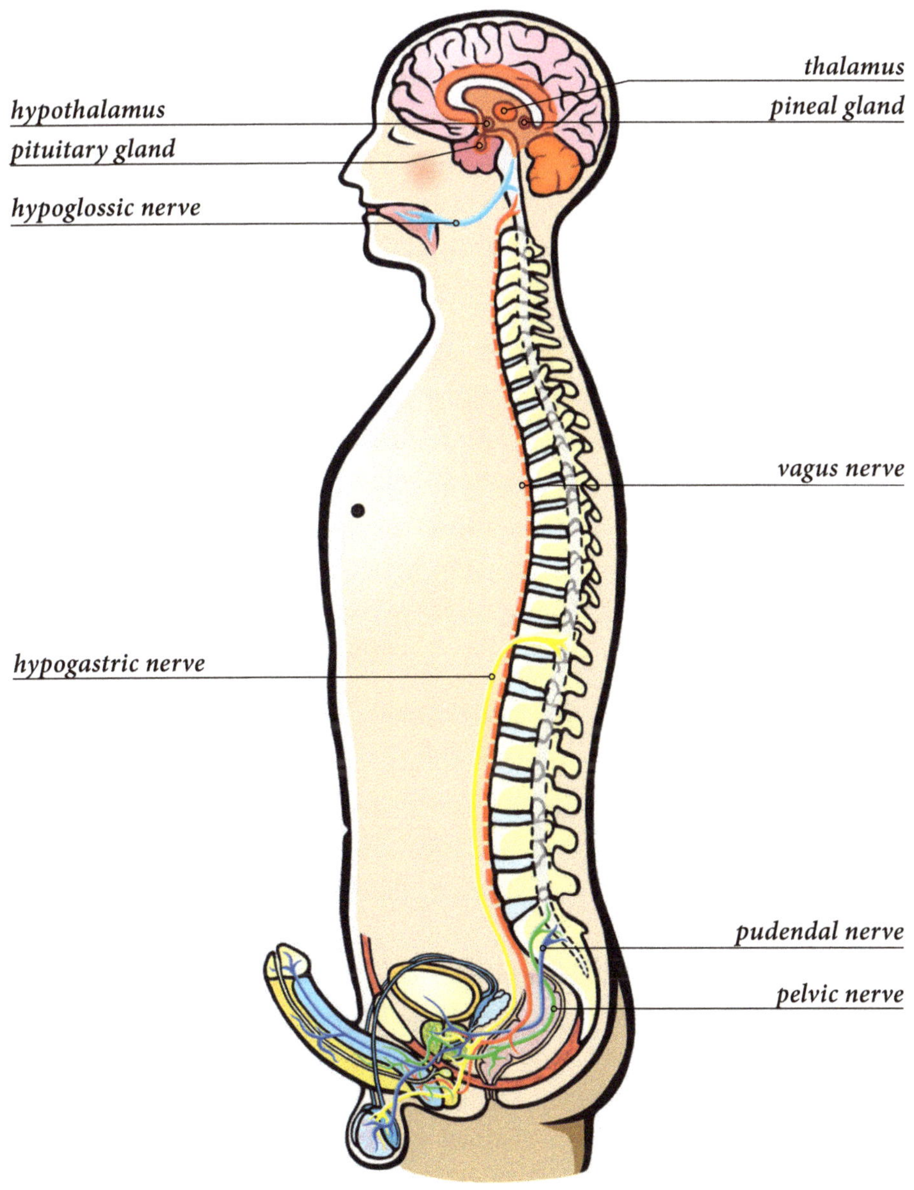

Your brain, nerves and genitals are intimately connected and affect eachother.

These are examples of how different parts of the body are connected, linked through the nerves and how they communicate with the brain. With new technology, it has been discovered that several parts of the brain are active before, during and after ejaculation and orgasm. The nerves interpret the sensual information through our senses and send signals to the brain, which increases or decreases the excitement. But it seems that the sum becomes much more than the parts. Scientific research still doesn't know how an orgasm is actually created.

Differences in the brain between men and women

There are several differences in the brain between men and women. Male brains are about 9% larger than female ones, but the number of brain cells is the same. The mesh in the brain that connects the cells with each other is different, female brains have more connections between the brain cells, which can also be seen in animals. In the end, everyone has the same abilities and qualities, but the underlying differences lead to slightly different ways of thinking and looking at the world. Men and women use different areas in the brain for problem solving, language processing, processing of experiences and for storing emotions. Women have greater brain space to process feelings and are generally better at expressing emotions and remembering details about emotional events. For example, men have 2.5 times as much brain space for sexual activity as well as larger brain centers for action and aggression. That men think more often about sex than women has been confirmed in many surveys. Brain research further shows that women need to feel comfortable and safe to want sex. The smallest occurrence can cause sexual disinterest. To feel safe, her foreplay therefore lasts 24 hours while his only lasts 3 minutes. When the estrogen (female sex hormone) takes over in the female brain, women begin to focus on their feelings and on communicating. As the testosterone flows into the body and brain of the man, they become obsessed with performing and get less likely to communicate. The examples are numerous and the list can be made long.

The point here is not to reinforce prejudice, but rather to inspire an increase in our understanding and respect for each other. Tao also talks about the fundamental differences between the essence of women and men and how it affects our way of interacting. Brain research seems to reflect this. Our gender roles appear to be a product of both biology and cultural influence as well as personal preferences.

In the book "The Female Brain" Louann Brizendine talks about how treacherous it is to pretending that women and men are the same and that the differences don't matter. There's nothing wrong with equality, but we just can't ignore the differences between men and women, because we often handle and process situations in different ways. On the other hand, we can increase our cohesion and thus the ability to understand and manage our differences, and similarities, in more creative and sensible ways. The differences in the brain are also not decisive for how we are, or to what degree we can educate ourselves, what talents we have, if we can engage with our children, if we like the same sex, or for our ability to create meaning in life or the development of our consciousness. We can all evolve by learning more about ourselves, and self-development is not a new concept. Tao has talked about human potential and our desire for self-realization for a long time. In the West, Freud and the psychological revolution were the first to claim that it was possible at all times to change our psyche. The latest brain research with the revolution of neurology also shows that the brain is much more malleable than we previously thought. It means you do not need to be the one you think you are, or have been so far. You can follow Tao's advice, instead of opposing change and new knowledge, choose to curiously explore different opportunities and put yourself in line with the change movement. Don't believe in anything, try it out to see if it works for you!

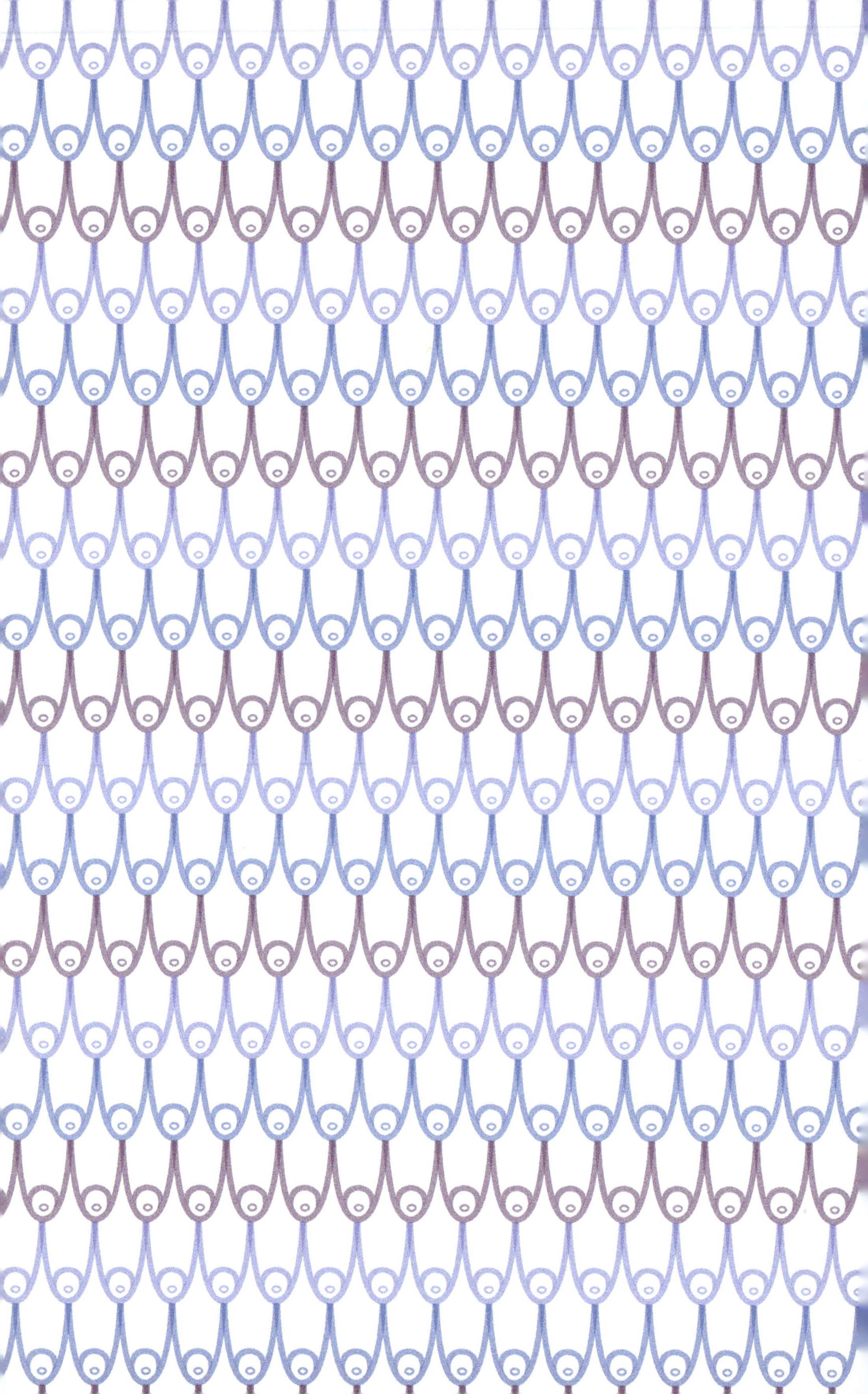

MALE
SEXUALITY

Why do we so rarely speak of male sexuality in positive and encouraging ways? Male sexuality has at times almost been demonized and portrayed as something more or less uncontrollable and potentially dangerous at its core. It is often portrayed to be uncomplicated, quick and unconscious. But male sexuality, just like female sexuality, is in it's foundation a positive energy. Besides from creating life it provides health, desire, pleasure, ecstasy and life energy. Male sexuality can also be sensitive and way more delicate than many believe. Female sexuality has often been presented as considerably more complex than the male one. Meter upon meter has been written about different points, zones and various female orgasms. The woman today is getting tips on how she can think positively about her sexuality and simultaneously take responsibility for herself, the same should apply to the men.

It is time for the men to reclaim a positive frame of mind regarding their sexuality. We need to create new symbolism and storys about the male potential, because even men have unheard of abilities within themselves. Knowledge about the male erotic potential and sensuality has existed for thousands of years in Eastern and Taoist wisdoms. Men have the same opportunities as women to vary and intensify their experience, and obtain full body orgasms as well as multiple orgasms.

Short is sweet

The arousal and excitement for men almost always ends with ejaculation. Most men have, what you call, a reasonable level of control over their ejaculation reflex. Studies show that the average time for sexual interaction is 5-7 minutes. Some men can extend the enjoyment to 15 minutes and a few up to 45 minutes. The obvious question is: how do those who can have longer intercourse do it? If you want to experience a sexuality where the whole body is filled with pleasure then, first of all, you need to keep it up for a long time. Obtaining ejaculation is certainly an intense pleasure in itself, but a few seconds of joy is difficult to compare with the feeling of timeless euphoria. This kind of well-being also strengthens health, brings new power and illuminates the soul. Instead of wasting your life energy, you can nourish yourself with it, as you will learn through the exercises further in the book.

Orgasm versus ejaculation

The orgasm is one of the most intense human experiences and it is different for different people and different for the individual. Among men it is common to connect orgasm with ejaculation and see them as inseparable. Within conventional medicine, the orgasm is seen as a reflex of muscular contractions in the pelvic floor which results in the release of seminal fluid. Here, the Taoist view differs from the conventional, and even newer Western research has found that an orgasm is about much more than a series of muscle contractions. When the body is stimulated, the lust center is activated in the brain, and vice versa. For example, you can have an orgasm in your sleep without touching the genitals. Stimulation of specific parts of the brain induces orgasm. Both men and women can imagine and fantasize their way to an orgasm. And it's not easy to explain how you have the ability to orgasm far earlier than your sexual maturity, even for children between the ages of two and three. It speaks for that the Taoists are right about the ability to separate the ejaculation from the orgasm. The orgasm is both a physical sensation, a strong feeling and an intense experience. It is both a biochemical phenomenon and an energy explosion.

> *When you have taught yourself to control "the point of no return" your pleasure reaches a far higher intensity and you may experience full body orgasm as well as multiple orgasms.*

Full body orgasm and multiple orgasms

The male pleasure is usually focused on the genitals. Wilhelm Reich (1897-1957), an Austrian psychoanalyst and student of Sigmund Freud, was the first from the West to claim that male orgasms include not only the genitals but the whole body. One of the fundamental principles you will learn from this book is the importance of separating the ejaculation from the orgasm. Just before the ejaculation, the emission occurs. That is when the sperm is mixed with other seminal fluids in the prostate. The second before the ejaculation, the widely known point of no return happens, the moment when it's too late to stop the ejaculation. You can learn to recognize the feeling that occurs even before the emission. The training then consists of halting the ejaculation but getting an orgasm. This will keep the erection and it is possible to get several orgasms in a row. You become multiorgasmic.

The sexual energy also needs help to be guided into the body and up the spine. Let the feeling you have in sex rise up the spine and spread throughout the body. As you master the technique of spreading and circulating the orgasmic feeling into the body, you can experience a full body orgasm. It can be described as several large waves instead of a single tsunami. You will be able to extend the intercourse and continue to be as turned on and orgasm over and over again. In the end, it's your own choice when it's time for ejaculation. The male's body has as great potential as women to have both full body orgasms and multiple orgasms. When you can enjoy and be stimulated for a longer time and have learned to not fall over the edge of point of no return then the enjoyment will increase in intensity. Just like women, men need to learn more about the phenomenon. They need to explore their body and discover, refine and manage these abilities.

A longtime Tao practitioner shares:

I had done a lot of yoga throughout the 80's. But it had not given me what I hoped about sexuality. Others recommended Mantak Chia and it was really great to meet him. There was not much talk about liberation on the one hand or to hold back the energy on the other hand. Mantak Chia said that if you do these exercises, your enjoyment will increase, while not losing energy. He also linked it to spirituality, a kind of spiritual training and personal development. I practiced intensively between 1993 and 2000. In the beginning I practiced a lot, sometimes 2-3 hours a day. The fact that sex was involved in part of the exercise made it only more rewarding. I have later expanded my training within Tao with other teachers. Today, I'm hesitant to just train the sexual energy. I don't think it works in depth. It is also about rediscovering what's hidden within us and where you need to advance in life. For exploring that, grounding in the physical body is important.

The exercises gave experiences similar to what I had with other spiritual teachers who did not work directly with the sexual energy. The training led me to control my ecstasy level and I could enter an ecstatic state at any time. It was a strength to be able to guide energy through the body to higher energy centers. After some time, I understood that the training would not give anything more than strong experiences if I didn't learn at the same time to build Qi in Dan Tian.

The strongest and most powerful insight was to realize that it is worth investing time in practice. It is fully possible to gain access to the body's ability to experience ecstasy and to have sex without losing energy. Other advantages are that if you have access to ecstasy, you don't need someone else to create it and can therefore be more present in the meeting with a partner. You can use the exercises only for sexual ecstasy and get high on it, but if you want to achieve deeper cultivation and build energy that stays, you should explore different ways in depth that fit one's purpose. The greatest has been to realize the profound understanding of life, which still lives within the various schools of Taoism, and so the real opportunities for development on all possible levels, which I, as a westerner, have not even dreamed of. Björn, 51 years old, kinesiologist and Qigong teacher

Ejaculation according to Tao

According to Tao, the man should learn to withhold his ejaculation. The reason is that he can make love for a longer time and generate energy instead of wasting it. It is well known that many men feel tired from "emptying" and the image of the man who empties and then turns around and falls asleep is too common. Immediate fatigue comes from building energy to quickly reach a climax and focusing on genitals and ejaculation. When this accumulation of excitement is released, the risk is great for a negative relaxation. Left behind is powerlessness and feelings of separation, apathy, irritation or emptiness.

By extending the enjoyment and delaying the timing of the ejaculation, you build up energy instead. When energy is generated in relaxation and awareness, it can expand and spread throughout the body. It creates satisfaction, strength and endurance as you retain the energy. By not ejaculating you have the opportunity to also use the energy of the sperm, especially if you also do the exercises from this book.

There are different perceptions about whether it is good to always stop the ejaculation. Many people think it is healthy to get a release on a regular basis. A measurement you can use is how energized you are after an ejaculation. Perhaps you are best off just ejaculating once a week or once a month? You need to learn what makes you feel good and recognize your own limits. Through energy exercises, you can also learn to absorb a lot of energy and not lose as much as you release. Especially if you learn to guide the energy through the spine and into the body. Increasing your stamina and prolonging the lovemaking has many advantages which everyone can enjoy.

In the classical Taoist texts about sex, men are recommended to ejaculate based on the formula: age x 0.2 = frequency. The recommendation will then be that at the age of 30, ejaculate at most every 6th day, at the age of 40 at the most every 8th day, at the age of 50 every 10 days etc. If you follow this advice, you can always make sure to replenish your own energy account and, in any case, not fall into the negative. However, the most important criterion is how your body feels. The sign of a good balance is that you feel comfortable, light and energized rather than lazy and sleepy after ejaculation. Of course, sex without ejaculation can be had more frequently.

The oral tradition within Tao also says that sex should be natural and not over-driven. Tao prefers neither to overtax the body with long sex marathons for several hours or to be fixed by always withholding your ejaculation, and thus having a bad conscience if you cross the line. Cultivating energy is about much more. When it comes to losing life energy, it's just as draining to be unsatisfied with your life and to live in self-denial.

Stopping the ejaculation

The easiest way to stop the ejaculation is by means of well-trained pelvic floor muscles. By squeezing around the mouth of the prostate just before the release, you can learn to master and prevent ejaculation. Instead of spilling, the sperm is recycled from the filled prostate and absorbed into the bloodstream. However, avoiding release by squeezing is not the same as fully mastering one's ejaculation. The difference lies in doing it in relaxation rather than effort. When you tense up, a need for discharge is created. Trying to push down or stall until you can't hold it anymore is a big effort. Therefore, that way of stopping ejaculation is not healthy in the long run. If you instead relax and guide the orgasmic energy up to the spine, ejaculation is eliminated by moving the focus away from the genitals and towards the brain, which reduces the excitement of the sex but increases the ecstatic feeling in the body.

Initially, exercise is about willpower and strengthening the pelvic floor muscles, but in the end it will be done through a soft squeeze, a thought and a clear intention. When you can prevent ejaculation during relaxation, the energy is built up and the excitement lasts longer. When the feeling approaches climax you relax even more and you let go of the hurry to ejaculate. This way energy is rebuilt over and over again. Once you allow yourself to come, you can do it fully and give in completely.

The start-stop method was launched by US sex therapist Helen Singer in the 1990s. It resembles Tao and is committed to learning to stay on a level of excitement where you can control the release. Further in this book you will find exercises where you practice this technique according to Tao. Take a look at the squeezing exercises and how to withhold the release.

Other methods to use in the heat of the moment are to pull out, so-called interrupted intercourse, or to simply hold for a few seconds. You can also ask your partner to squeeze hard around the penis at the edge where the glans begins, or do so yourself. The Tao also advocates moving slowly and not going too fast during lovemaking in order to feel more and stay sensitive, which allow man to make love longer and lessen his need to ejaculate. In addition, an approach that will be appreciated by many women. Over time, you will find that the automatic urge to ejaculate will begin to reside.

The Million dollar spot

Within Tao, there is another technique to stop ejaculation called the million dollar spot. The name predicts the high value of preserving the sperm. By pressing the million dollar spot in the perineum (see p. 137), it is possible to prevent the release. The method is to use the three middle fingers and push hard enough, but not so hard that it hurts, to prevent the sperm from getting out of the prostate into the urethra. Press the middle of the perineum a few seconds before and during the orgasm. It is important to learn to find the right spot. If you press too close to the anus, the release is not blocked, and if you push too close to the scrotum, it ends up in the urine. In both cases, you lose the benefits.

If you want to use the million dollar spot, it is recommended that you do energy or Qigong exercises to guide the energy further into your body. Otherwise, you only block the release physically and no transformation occurs, which in the long run can cause imbalances. If you have problems with the prostate, the recommendation is to not use the million dollar spot.

Premature ejaculation

The perhaps biggest problem for a man is not to be able to control his ejaculation. About 40% of all men between 18-74 years old in Sweden have sporadically experienced early ejaculation and around 10% experience that they always have it. Exactly where the limit goes for being called "premature ejaculation" is hard to say. Some criteria are that the intercourse lasts less than 2 minutes, that the man is not in control and that it's perceived as a problem. At the same time, that figure can be compared to the average time of intercourse in western Europe, which is about 5-7 minutes. Premature ejaculation is most common in younger men. The men who suffer from premature ejaculation don't have, for various reasons, the ability of control. They get release as soon as they reach a certain level of excitement, whether they want to or not. This can of course create frustration and disappointment in intimate situations. You are not born with the ability to postpone your ejaculation, you must conquer it. The release reflexes are controlled by the sympathetic nervous system, acting independently and beyond our control. Nevertheless, you can influence the outcome by affecting the parasympathetic nervous system, which activates when you relax.

Reasons for premature ejaculation

Premature ejaculation can have many different causes and occur in different contexts. The reason can be neurological, biochemical, psychological or social. Physical illness, medication, religious or cultural condition, shame, depression, low self-esteem and stress can affect it. Some men may have developed early release through the fear of being discovered when they masturbated early in life. Others may have had bad experiences from different partners who have triggered a negative pattern. The phenomenon may also vary in different situations, for example, whether you are by yourself or if you are with someone. Being in love, nervousness during intercourse and perceived demands for a union can be very stressful for a man. Another underlying cause of premature ejaculation may be a weak prostate, or weak or constantly tense pelvic floor muscles. Men with inadequate control of ejaculation do have problems with their sexual self-esteem and may unfortunately be reluctant to talk about their sexual problems. Many men tend to underestimate the psychological stressors and find it hard to see the connection to a physical symptom like premature ejaculation. The famous flight or fight reflex makes it so that the blood leaves the genitals within seconds.

Perhaps it's sometimes an all-natural reaction to a certain situation to have a premature ejaculation, or failure to have an erection for that matter. It may be the body's own way of communicating what you need. Maybe your feelings are not in flow and you try to hold back something that creates an inner stress. Vulnerability, insecurity or something delicate wants to come through. In this way, the body becomes a messenger for how to balance your emotional aspect and it becomes a matter of how to integrate your experience. You can meet the situation by just being with what is and letting what wants to happen to happen. You then become aware of yourself and can express what you need in the moment. The unpleasant emotion transforms into vitality and increases your awareness.

Whatever reasons for the problems, the exercises in this book provide you with the opportunity to develop both a connection with your emotions and relaxation of the body. You will learn how to strengthen the pelvic floor muscles and also how to make them relax. You train yourself to focus inward and find out how you work and how you want things. By getting to know yourself, you create security. Being conscious of bodily sensations and having the courage to communicate your thoughts and feelings provides the best conditions for creating a healthy and fruitful sex life.

Treatment for premature ejaculation

There is a wide range of quick solutions to premature ejaculation, ranging from anesthetic spray and penis rings to trying to think of something "boring". To masturbate and come once before intercourse and reduce arousal is another "quick fix". A Taoist method to prevent premature ejaculation during intercourse is to relax the pelvic floor just as you slip into the vagina and squeeze when you withdraw. Tao also speaks of individual cultivation of the sexual energy. You practice to postpone the ejaculation and spread the aroused feeling. By changing your focus you can learn how to control the excitement. After you have prolonged the pleasure and repeated this behavior, the sexual reaction eventually becomes automated. Then you don't have to exert yourself as much to have control. Instead, you can focus on relaxing and enjoying sex on a more intense level. As already mentioned, it is also about regaining a connection with your emotional life and recreating a healthy relationship with yourself.

Impotence

To get an erection requires interplay between the nervous system, blood vessels and the hormone system and between thoughts and feelings. There can be many causes of impotence and often there are several factors that interact. The problem is similar to the premature ejaculation. Tao associates impotence primarily with a failing prostate or imbalance in the kidney Qi. Stress or nervousness is another common, often underestimated, cause of erection failure. In stress, anxiety or worry, the body excretes stress hormones that inhibit blood flow to the penis. All power goes to the extremities, arms and legs, to prepare for flight, fight or playing dead. Within a few seconds, the swelling bodies in the penis will drain of blood and relax. Impotence can also be related to boring or a routine of sex. Being tender and loving towards your own body, or allowing your partner to be, can be a way of creating security and building self-esteem. Allowing only to receive can be redeeming and awaken new lusts. Through loving unconditional touch of the entire body, the ability to enjoy it comes back

Masturbation

Basically all men masturbate and it is a natural act, and most do it throughout their lives and whether they have a partner or not. Some men worry about if they masturbate too often. Different cultures have always had different views on masturbation, it has often been condemnatory, including in Taoism. There it has been condemnatory about the "usual" way of masturbating: by stimulating penis for ejaculation of semen and letting the energy go to waste. You also risk over stimulating an organ because different parts of the penis are linked to different organs in the body. The heart zone is closest to the penis head and is easiest to stimulate to orgasm. The heart becomes over-stimulated while the other internal organs are underpinned. You should therefore avoid stimulating only a portion of the penis. Instead, give the whole penis as much attention and train yourself to prolong the pleasure and, if you want, to hold back the release, but get an orgasm A slight change in your habit will pay off..

Circumcision

Cutting off the foreskin on the penis head is common in many places in the world. The circumcision often has religious or cultural connotations, but also for hygienic and physical reasons. Sometimes the procedure is carried out at an early age and sometimes on the young man as a transitional rite into the adult world. For all men it is important to keep clean around the foreskin where bacteria can easily thrive. If you are circumcised, sometimes the sensitivity may have decreased if nerve endings are damaged. On the other hand, it probably means you can last longer. Though some experience that the sensitivity of the exposed glans increases.

The male burden to perform

Many men would give their right hand to know how to be a good man and a good lover. Whether you are aware of it or not, your identity and self-image is based upon how you perceive yourself as a sexual being - your genital sense of self. This leads to high demands on sexual performance. Sometimes, to a large extent, it becomes impossible to be present and relax. Many men are so busy with trying to be perfect lovers and being afraid to fail and to be criticized that they almost miss the pleasure along the way. Others have developed a strong sexual control that leads to a fear of losing oneself. You are never good enough and think you need more discipline. The quest to be perfect never ends. There are reports of sixteen year-olds in Sweden who take Viagra to be sure to perform as well as possible. This can not be the right way.

In addition, there are many men who feel obliged to satisfy the woman. Sometimes this stress is temporarily buried in a comfortable working sexual routine. Not being accepted and recognized as a good lover can be very difficult for a man to deal with. His whole manhood is at stake. In order to be able to relax, he needs to get rid of the idea that he is 100% responsible for the result of the love making. It's not just the man's responsibility to make sure the loving is going well, there's just as much responsibility for the woman.

Men often lack valuable knowledge of what is important in close relationships and are unable to be present and intimate. Instead, unrealistic demands and expectations are imposed on the relationship. Feelings live in the body and you can practice recognizing bodily sensations and emotional sensations, in order to become more aware of your needs. The meditations and exercises further contribute to increasing this sensitivity and awareness.

The breath is the bridge to the inside

Breathing acts like a bridge between the body and your feelings. Through breathing you can touch the inner you and help the body relax. If you don't have a connection with your body, you are also not aware of how you really feel. When your breathing is irregular, fast and up in the chest, it is easy to lose contact with your inner guide. In a stressed situation, it helps to breathe deeply, rhythmically and slowly. Conscious breathing balances emotions and helps a stressed brain to wind down. Breathe quietly, through the nose, into the stomach and with a smooth rhythm. A relaxed body and upright posture makes it easier to maintain a rhythmic, deep and calm breath. Make it a habit of always being aware of your breathing, not just in the exercises, and let it guide you towards a clearer connection and deeper relaxation, so you can be present in your body and with your feelings.

Feelings and sex

When you begin to explore your sexuality, what often happens is that old feelings, memories or experiences associated with early experiences of sex will appear. There might be feelings of shame around masturbation, criticism from an early girlfriend or comparisons with other men. The general attitude of Tao towards emotions, which gets their fuel from past events, is that they are all there for a good reason, but they need to be flowing and balanced. What is repressed doesn't disappear by itself over time, it continues to affect us without us being aware of it. Feelings also become a filter as we look through the world and we project our shortcomings onto others. Without being conscious, we repeat the same pattern over and over again. Whether you're living out dramas and dumping your energy on others, or have shut off unpleasant feelings and closed them off, they hurt you. Part of the solution is to get to know the thoughts and attitudes behind them and become aware of the inner dialogue. You need to be honest with yourself and perceive what views you defend to create the inner conflict. As humans we are still maturing emotionally. We make feelings too personal. Part of the process is changing our focus and taking a more neutral standpoint. Try the exercise on p. 105-106 on the intelligence of the heart.

As long as unhealthy trauma, shame and blame is in the way, sexuality can not be expressed naturally. Societal values about male sexuality have not promoted a natural and neutral attitude. By honoring and accepting your feelings, no matter what form they are taking at the moment, you will continue forward.

Let's do a small test by examining the shame you're wearing. Pick a memory from an embarrassing situation. Do you notice how the shame remains and that it is difficult to accept the feeling? Instead of approaching the feeling, you begin to defend yourself by thinking of something else, criticizing yourself or judging the other person. In other words, you try to be something you are not, the sense of shame prevents you from being authentic. Living in honesty and truth and walking the path of your heart requires that you allow yourself to become aware of what you deny and then identify the cause. What do you really feel? If you don't feel what you feel, you can't obtain the information and you'll mislead yourself. You lose contact with both your real needs and your true intuition. See your feelings of discomfort or vulnerability as a path to potential wisdom and renewed strength. Nobody is perfect and everyone has weaknesses.

> *Sex is not just an external activity, but an inner experience of being.*

Perhaps you are afraid to be seen in a bad way or to show yourself vulnerable? Perhaps you feel unfairly treated and not entitled to stand up for yourself? Or do you have strong forbidden feelings and fantasies that are difficult to handle? Our own fear of failure and to fit in, and the cultural clichés surrounding that, hold us in our old ways. When feelings of shame are displaced to the unconscious, they can appear as perversions or inhibition instead. If you have trouble getting out of a negative pattern or old negative behaviors, seek professional help. Being mirrored by a neutral and professional person can be illuminating and of great value.

Sex and heart

To withhold ejaculation can trigger unexpected reactions. Controlling behavior or vulnerability suddenly surface. That's because you start to open yourself up, and feelings come forth and that's good. It's part of your development and creates the opportunity to get in touch with your real needs and the desire of your heart. Allow yourself to feel and embrace yourself. Feel the deep relaxation in acknowledging that you are good just the way you are. When the heart opens up and your feelings are balanced, your genitals will also be filled with a strong and loving feeling. A willingness to receive yourself and a desire to give love takes shape. This feeling grows and fills the heart with self-esteem and happiness. When you can accommodate a larger spectrum of your emotional life, you can maintain strong feelings without losing yourself, and even affirm the more subtle intuitive feelings without neglecting them. It is through emotions and love we come alive. This will affect your way of relating as well as your orgasms.

Exhibitionism and voyeurism

The fact that men like watching the woman is not news, nor that the woman likes to hear compliments and that this may raise an interest in each other. Vision can be the gateway to other feelings for the man, while hearing can indirectly raise feelings for the woman. Interestingly, within the "five element theory" of Chinese medicine, male sexuality is linked to the liver whose sense is the sight - to look and project. The female sexuality is connected to the kidneys, whose sense is the hearing - to listen and to take in. Both men and women can enjoy taking both positions. You can be voyeuristic and allow yourself to really watch and look at your partner, and give appreciation, or be the exhibitionist, the one who enjoys inviting the watcher and being looked at, and receive fully. This strengthens the intimacy, and in addition to the willingness to explore, also requires caution and respect for each other. No one wants to just be an object or hear words without substance.

Sexual desire

The more you seek sensations, the less sensitive you will be. Perhaps we have never been so insensitive and as numb as we are today. An increasing number of young men are witnessing the so-called "porn impotence", which means that they can be erect when they look at porn, but not with their woman. Online flow of information is enormous and access to instructions and tips about sex and porn is endless. Nevertheless, the sex tips in the media is quite stereotypical; they are often about external solutions with suggestions for new sex toys, new places, new positions or new creams and pills. But will all this lead to pleasure in the long-term or changes in depth over time? Sex is not just an external activity, but an inner experience and a journey.

When our feelings are blurred, stronger stimuli are required to make us feel. In order to increase the intensity of sensations, we must increase the pace, increase the frequency of movement, change partners, watch more porn etc. The need to do more to compensate when we feel less never ends. Then it becomes this mechanical repetition which removes us from our feelings and sensitivity. Some call it "rubbing" or "friction sex", as we just keep going by masturbating ourselves or each other. As soon as something becomes mechanical, the unconsciousness has emerged, and thus the lack of presence and sensitivity is a fact. We become incapable of experiencing ourselves with some major meaning. We become climax machines. When sex is reduced to an easy lay, we lose contact with the deepest being of sexuality. But why the rush? Take time instead to enjoy the view, listen to the love expressions, feel the smells and above all feel deeper inside the body and further into the soul. Allow yourself to follow through all the way into the core of your origins and receive both yourself, your partner and the mutual creative power. Being here and now and feeling more - big emotions as well as subtle sensations - create sensuality and more lust.

To be, not to do

In Tao and Tantra, sex is more about being than doing. It's a misconception to believe that the more you do, the more pleasant sex becomes. On the contrary, the less you do and the more you relax, the more you feel. Sexual ecstasy goes hand in hand with calmness, deep breathing and physical relaxation. Relaxation is the opposite of performance, effort and tension. This is the same for both men and women. Unconsciously, we have become accustomed to focusing on the future, on climax, on orgasm. If you are focused on what will happen later you are not present. Keeping the attention of the moment will generate relaxation and focus on the meeting. The strange thing is how much energy there is and how much energy can arise from stillness and awareness. Try to be completely still the next time you make love. You will have a positive surprise. Being more than doing does not mean that the love making can't be varied and both hard and soft and fast and slow. The difference is that the different movements do not arise from a thought but come from being present. The receptivity to the energy movement creates a natural spontaneity. So be open to trying new grips, it's ok to "mess up" and learn from your mistakes. That's when you stop focusing on the next goal and doing something "right" and you become responsive, creative and inventive. Spontaneity gives you experiences and insights that guide you to the nature and safety of your presence.

A woman describes a meeting:

For a period I was together with a very responsive and receptive man. It was both playful and magical. Our love meetings began with our senses being activated, our joy to see each other, a soft conversation, the smell of excitement pheromones and then the feeling and taste of each other's bodies. I noticed that he had been training on the touch and massage of different parts of the body, from the face and the breasts to the labia and the zones inside. He had a complete awareness of his penis and made use of the muscles and was able to decide when to come or when to be still. At the same time, he was receptive and present. The rhythm varied, slowly sometimes and faster sometimes. He followed my rhythm and could build my orgasm. For every orgasm I climbed higher and higher. He could also relax himself and be with me in the aftermath and follow when it increased again. I felt a tremendous connection with him and between us. Even though I didn't actively practice, for example, the small circulation, I could feel how energy circulated in the body, through all chakras. Especially when I sat in his lap, I could feel it. We sat still and breathed and everything just flowed. He could orgasm without ejaculating. It is such a beautiful memory.

It can be hard to understand that there may be something beyond normal sex if you never got in touch with it. You have to open your eyes to see the light, you have to believe that you can. Some men react with performance anxiety when they hear of something like this, and others say YES, guide me! Techniques, however, are nothing unless the connection is available. The how is more important than the what.

Karin, teacher, 49 years old

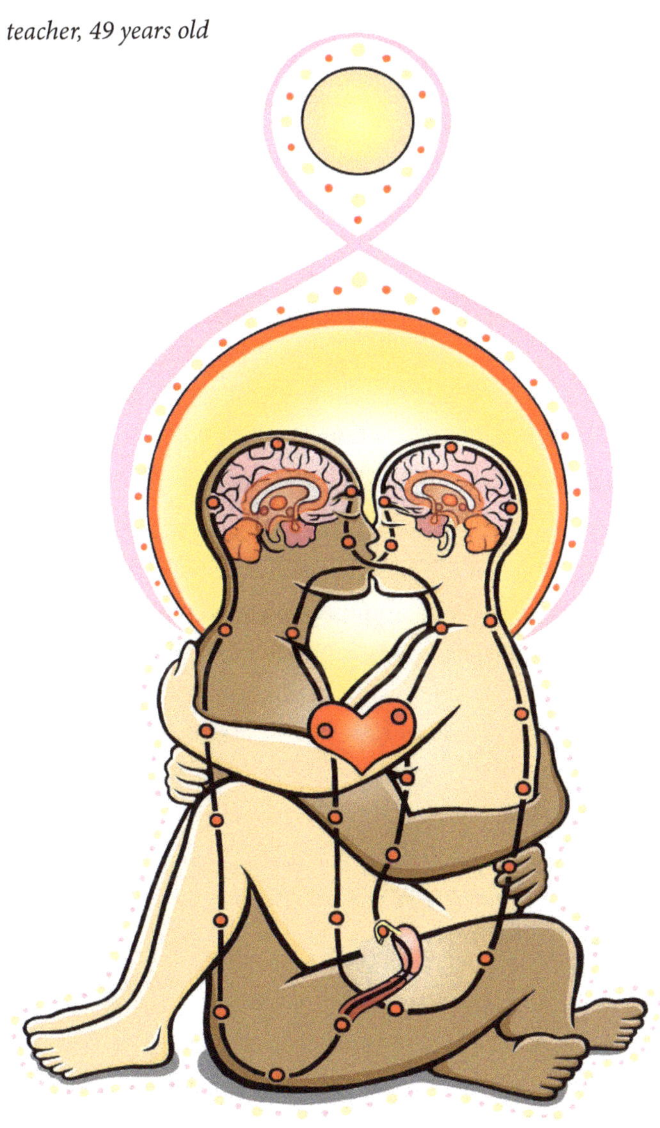

Cultivation with a partner and circulating the energies between each other.

Different types of orgasms

Nowadays, several types of orgasms are also known for men, such as penile orgasm, P-zone orgasm, mixed orgasm, (both penis and P-zone), full body orgasm (sometimes called energy orgasm) and multiple orgasms (several in a row). There are different levels depending on how the energy is rising in your body and affects your chakras. With focus solely on the genitals, the energy only rises to the first chakra. If it rises through the spine and out into the body, you keep energy and the experience becomes completely different. The orgasm may be explosive or flowing, short or long, weak or strong and may occur with or without ejaculation. The most healthy and rewarding thing ought to be getting different types of orgasms.

No matter what pleasure zone you stimulate or what kind of orgasm you get, you learn in the Taoist exercises to lift the sexual energy and spread the orgasmic power through your chakras and into the body. The effect of moving the energy upwards is unexplored here in the west but well known in Tao, Quodoushka and Tantra. There, sexual energy is associated not only with good health but also with a long life of joy and with the exploration of other worlds. Actually, it is weird that this most satisfying ability we have received is so unexplored in our culture. It is as if we expect the knowledge about sex life to be there by itself. Unfortunately, it's not always that way. But as with so much else, it is knowledge, understanding and practice which provide skills.

Directing the energy inward and upward along the channel in your spine helps it reach the pituitary gland and the pineal gland, endocrine glands in the brain. With these we control and create our erotic and creative expressions. The ability to guide energy in combination with relaxation, deep breath, bodily awareness, presence, consciousness, will, feeling, love, open heart and ability to let go of control and engage yourself creates different levels of intensity in your orgasm. A clear sign that you moved and gained energy from the sexual meeting or an orgasm is that you feel alert and awake afterwards.

Orgasm through the P-zone

The male's equivalent to the woman's G-zone is called the P-zone. It is the prostate, which is an erotic body, in both sexes, and is sensitive to stimulus. You can stimulate it through perineum or anus. When the prostate is stimulated via the anus, some men usually describe it as a more protracted sense of lust where the ejaculate rather flows than sprays out. The prostate is emptied slowly and the orgasm may take several minutes. The experience is similar to the differences that women express about G-zone and clitoral stimulation. Different nerves give rise to different experiences. P-zone orgasms can also be done without ejaculation. Many men experience great pleasure with a prostate orgasm, especially with both prostate and penis stimulation at the same time.

Olivier, 44, talks about his experience of prostate stimulation via anus:

It was a different input and a more direct and uncontrollable feeling. I felt more vulnerable, the "masculine" energy came in and I had to get more receptive and open to let it in. To me, it was also about opening a "closed symbol" to dare to try something which was previously forbidden. My experience of the actual orgasm was not very different from usual.

Different orgasmic expressions

There are different aspects of the man as a lover where his natural essence is expressed. It is a delusion to just have one image of the male orgasmic expression, as a strong erection with a powerful spray. Within the shamanic love art and book Quodoushka (Amara Charles), several different variations of male orgasmic expressions are described.

For example, you can experience a strong orgasm with a flaccid penis that fully ejaculates, especially when you are intimate with strong feelings for a partner. The orgasm slowly builds up, comes unexpectedly, and is like waves of emotion with a focus on the heart. Sometimes mistaken as premature ejaculation.

Another type of orgasm is when you focus simultaneously on the genitals and the head. The arousal is strong and perhaps inspired by erotic words or fantasies. When the point of no return approaches, you relax all the muscles of your body, especially in the pelvis, while you breathe deep into your stomach, in the same rhythm as your orgasm. This is most similar to what the Tao speaks of, a full orgasm without ejaculation, with an erect penis. A pleasure that relieves stress and leaves you peaceful with clarity in your mind.

Furthermore, Quodoushka describes a type of orgasm where you have a full erection and you get full release. You give yourself fully with a strong focus on the genitals. The movement comes from deep within, like an earthquake, and the body shakes from pleasure. Afterwards you feel comfortable and you are filled with new healthy energy, provided that the energy is guided up in the body.

There is also an orgasm without erection and without spray. When waves of love rise from the genitals, which then spread into the body. Some men describe it as an electric current, which comes like fast, hot flames. This is a gift which broadens awareness and brings a sense of freedom and happiness. Jens, 59, describes this:

For me, it happens in long erotic meetings when the entire body is aroused. Then the fire comes suddenly, my body gets hot, the skin gets prickly from the heat and I'm burning. Flaccid cock and no ejaculation, but an expansion of joy and pure love.

Perhaps this only sounds remarkable and impossible to manage. It's not supposed to discourage you, but rather to inspire and tell you about different possibilities. The keys to getting into the different experiences are to relax into the enjoyment and let go of all your fantasies, expectations and goals, and go where your energy guides you. One tip is to follow the woman's energy in sexual encounters, because she has a tendency to be a step ahead. When you manage to release control, spontaneously new and unforeseen events and experiences occur. They are an expression of your masculine essence and the inherent nature of the body. Getting different types of orgasms helps you to expand your life experience and it prepares the way to become a more mature and balanced person in the new era of gender equality and cooperation.

Become a better lover

Wanting to be a better lover begins well before the act of love itself. Everything you think, say and do accumulate within you. Either you create relaxation and harmony, or you build tensions and inner contradictions. It's all about your life, not just things that have to do with sex. Examples of things that create internal tension are a white lie, unconscious denials or a simple but important feeling that is not communicated. That you do something you really cannot stand for or compromise yourself. Internally you may bear these shortcomings and you become more vulnerable. Internal contradictions also sit inside the body and it becomes tense and uncomfortable. Instead of being present, you are busy being on guard and defending yourself. This does not benefit you as a love partner. In the long term, the internal stress created can have devastating consequences. No matter how terrible we think we are and what we have done before or how impossible the conflicts are, it is acceptance and honesty that pave the way for a life, and above all a love life, in harmony.

The power of words

To start verbalizing your feelings and to be honest is liberating. Words have a magical power to be released when expressed in the present, while being linked to your truth and your feelings. The frozen inner images melt and become flowing vitality. Words of humor can promote healthy distance and liberate a locked or embarrassing situation. Words are important to affect, create contact and intimacy. It is by sharing your feelings that you communicate and give appreciation and love. It is through them you create intimate lasting relationships.

Tips from women

All women are different. Both anatomy and mind vary, which means that a technique or a way to seduce, which has worked with one woman may not work at all with another. Some women are quickly physically turned on while others need more emotional confirmation first. Others get turned on by intellectual stimulus or imagination and some want to feel spiritually inspired. All these preferences also vary on different occasions for every single woman. Nevertheless, here are some general tips about women.

A woman wants to feel sought after, loved and appreciated. She appreciates your mental radiance and that you are open hearted in your communication. She wants to feel your heart and at the same time your desire. She wants to feel your eyes, your hands, your body and your limb. She wants you to know what you want, but at the same time that you can be responsive to her different needs. She wants to be seen and feel safe. For the woman, it is important that there is a connection before you can even think about exploring her body. Her foreplay begins in that sense well before the actual act. It is important to her that you are clear and responsive, as well as to be clear on what feelings and chemistry there is between you.

Breasts are central to a woman's experience of ecstasy and is often the safest way to a woman's love, interest and devotion. They are her plus pole and are directly connected to both the heart and the genitals. In practice, this means that from the beginning the breasts are more important than her genitals. Through stimulation, hormones are secreted that open up the vagina and increase her receptivity. When a loving emphasis is placed on her breasts before penetration, it facilitates her arousal. But keep in mind that all women experience their breasts in different ways. For those women whose breasts have not been handled carefully or have not been appreciated and cared for, it may take some time to feel pleasure. A physical, loving touch without demands causes the oxytocin and the sense of togetherness to flow. So take it easy in the beginning and learn to give and receive touch with full attendance. Many also want and need eye contact and kisses to get turned on.

> *Acceptance and honesty pave the way for a life, and above all a love life, in harmony.*

Let her show you how she wants it and teach her how to stimulate you. Do what you do because you like doing it, not because you're going to achieve something or are going somewhere. Find your partner's enjoyment and keep in mind that she needs to be fully turned on before you penetrate her. That means she is wet, moves and sounds. It's a betrayal of love if the woman is forced into the sex act before she's open and ready. If this happens continuously for several years, the woman will certainly tire and eventually refuse sex. Ask her to invite you when she's ready. Then you don't have to worry about when the right moment to approach her comes. Enter her slowly and take time to really feel, not just the tip of the penis, but the whole penis, and then your entire body. If the woman and her vagina are fully turned on when you enter, it can lead to a different experience of sex. An electromagnetic potential occurs, like in the attraction between two magnets. This awakens what some call Kundalini energy, which, according to Tantra, is symbolized by the ascending snake of the masculine, which then implodes in the feminine. Some describe this experience as "ultimate spirituality". According to Tao, it's a love act where you share each other's essence, the woman absorbs your yang and you her yin. This exchange, as well as circulating energy, is the essence of the Taoist love making.

If you want to make love for a long time and bring you and your partner to new heights, a hot tip is to slow down and cool down the mood for a while. She needs to understand that she should not concentrate on your climax. It is common for women to require a "receipt" that the sex act has been good. Many women think they are not loved or attractive if the man does not come. Therefore, you must tell her that it feels okay for you anyway.

If you want to avoid ejaculation, make sure that the love making becomes slow and sensual, with less of the rough stimulus and eager arousal from the beginning. Help her relax deeper. Relax into your body, into the pelvic floor and focus on your own heart. But, if you feel you cross the limit, tell your woman that you need to come, look her in the eyes, stay present in the situation, let go and enjoy.

Keep in mind that you can not demand to deposit your semen in the woman if she doesn't approve of it. Request permission or agree before where the release should end up. You can not assume that she uses any protection. The easiest and best way to take responsibility for unwanted pregnancies is to use a condom, which also provides protection against sexually transmitted diseases. No ejaculation is also no guarantee that it doesn't transmit sperm cells into the love fluids. Respect and responsibility for each other belongs to love. It may also be appropriate to take it easy with the practice of "exercises" during the act, partly because it is a strong force and partly because the woman usually does not appreciate when the man is "going at it", which often happens at the expense of presence in the meeting. The intimate room is a delicate presence that requires conscious care and consideration.

Female anatomy

An investigation by RFSU, "Swedish Association for Sexual Education", showed that 58% did not know how big a clitoris is. It was a web survey answered by 1,000 men and women between 18-45 years. This may not be strange since it was only in the late 1990s that it became clear that the woman's clitoris consists of erectile tissue of about 4 inches which, like penises, swell upon excitement. However, only the clitoral head is visible, which has double the amount of nerve endings that the male glans has.

Another of the female's erotic zones is the G-zone. It is the female prostate, which is a sensitive area and an erectile tissue around the urethra. Like the man's prostate it contains glands that hold ejaculate. You can feel the beginning of the prostate body, as a meaty area, around the urethral opening. Further in it feels like a weakly grooved area, about 1-2 inches in on the vagina's front wall, closest to the stomach. This is the place where most women experience the pleasurable G-zon. In some women, the G-zone is rather far in and is therefore inaccessible with the fingers.

The A-zone is a sensitive area far into the vagina, almost up by the cervix, toward the front vaginal wall. The cervix itself is also an erogene zone in women, but it needs to be approached gently, softly and with awareness - it should not hurt. Actually, intercource should never hurt, not even the first time.

The experience of the different erotic zones varies from woman to woman. Some have a lot of experience and have explored themselves, others have not. But most can learn to enjoy more.

A woman has several erotic flows from different glands, which make the vagina soft and wet. It has also been found that most women ejaculate during sexual activity, though often in small amounts. The female ejaculate comes from the female prostate gland and contains similar substances as the man's, with the exception of semen. There is also a phenomenon called squirting. Whilst doing so, the woman sprays a greater amount of ejaculate. For a full description of the female anatomy as well as erotic zones and flows, read more in my book about women's sexual well-being.

Another remarkable result of RFSU's survey was that 55% of men believe that women easiest get pregnant two to three days before her period. That's not correct. The easiest time to become pregnant for women would be about two weeks after the first day of menstruation. Then ovulation lasts for about three days. The sperm can survive up to five days inside the vagina. The woman can take the temperature of and feel her secretion to know exactly when she ovulates. Today, there are also various methods and tests to buy at the pharmacy that helps keep track of the fertile days.

What happens in the meeting?

According to the RFSU survey, 65% believe that it is the physical conditions that make it take longer for women to get an orgasm. The general attitude also seems to be that it takes longer for a woman than a man to get turned on. Even the Tao talks about how the woman being water and the man fire, and that it takes longer to "warm up" the water than to speed up the fire. That may be true, but in masturbation there is no difference. It seems to be in the meeting of people where it changes. In fact, in the well-known Kinsey-survey from the 1950s, when 6,000 American women were interviewed, it was found that half of all women were masturbating and 90% could take themselves to an orgasm in less than 3 minutes! The conclusion must be that it is in the meeting with a partner that something happens. So what's happening in our relationships?

The figure that an average sexual intercourse lasts for 5-7 minutes is derived from a study conducted in 2008. The survey is based on responses from experienced psychologists, physicians and therapists who have found that the average sexual intercourse lasts 3-13 minutes. Since women are more naturally focused on intimacy and love, and often able to enjoy longer, the love making may be less interesting to her if the man has difficulty being present in the meeting and instead focus on performance. The woman might also tire if during this short period of time, you only focus on the genitals and mechanical sex without emotional attachment. With repeated unsatisfactory meetings, the woman's body slowly and gradually shuts off. She feels unsuccessful and unhappy. This happens especially if the sex is always overheated, fast and hard. In order to be ready and open up her love gates, the woman, as we have already seen, needs contact, safety, appreciation and presence.

Another important ingredient for creating fruitful relationships may be to have a clearly expressed intention with the meeting or relationship. Why do you want to meet? Relationship? Sex? Explore different things or roles? The agreement provides a clear framework for the meeting which guides both intentions and strengthens security. It also works as an antidote against unspoken and unrealistic expectations of a meeting or a relationship. Hopes that in the worst case it only causes misunderstandings, separation and unhappiness.

The fact that the basic sexuality of the man and woman is different is not strange. Physically and physiologically, it is obvious. One sex is outgoing and fertilizes, the other is inward, is fertilized and gives birth. Ecstasy means to "go out of yourself" to meet what's different. The word sex comes from "secare" and initially means to distinguish, which indicates polarity. The man enjoys the woman and the woman enjoys the man. Tao believes that the woman's gift to the man is to make him open up his heart while the man's gift for the woman is to help her to open up sexually. We all have the polarities inside of us, it's just that we start on opposite ends. It's the differences, also regardless of gender, that give richness and inspiration and create the attraction. In the next chapter we explore the masculine essence.

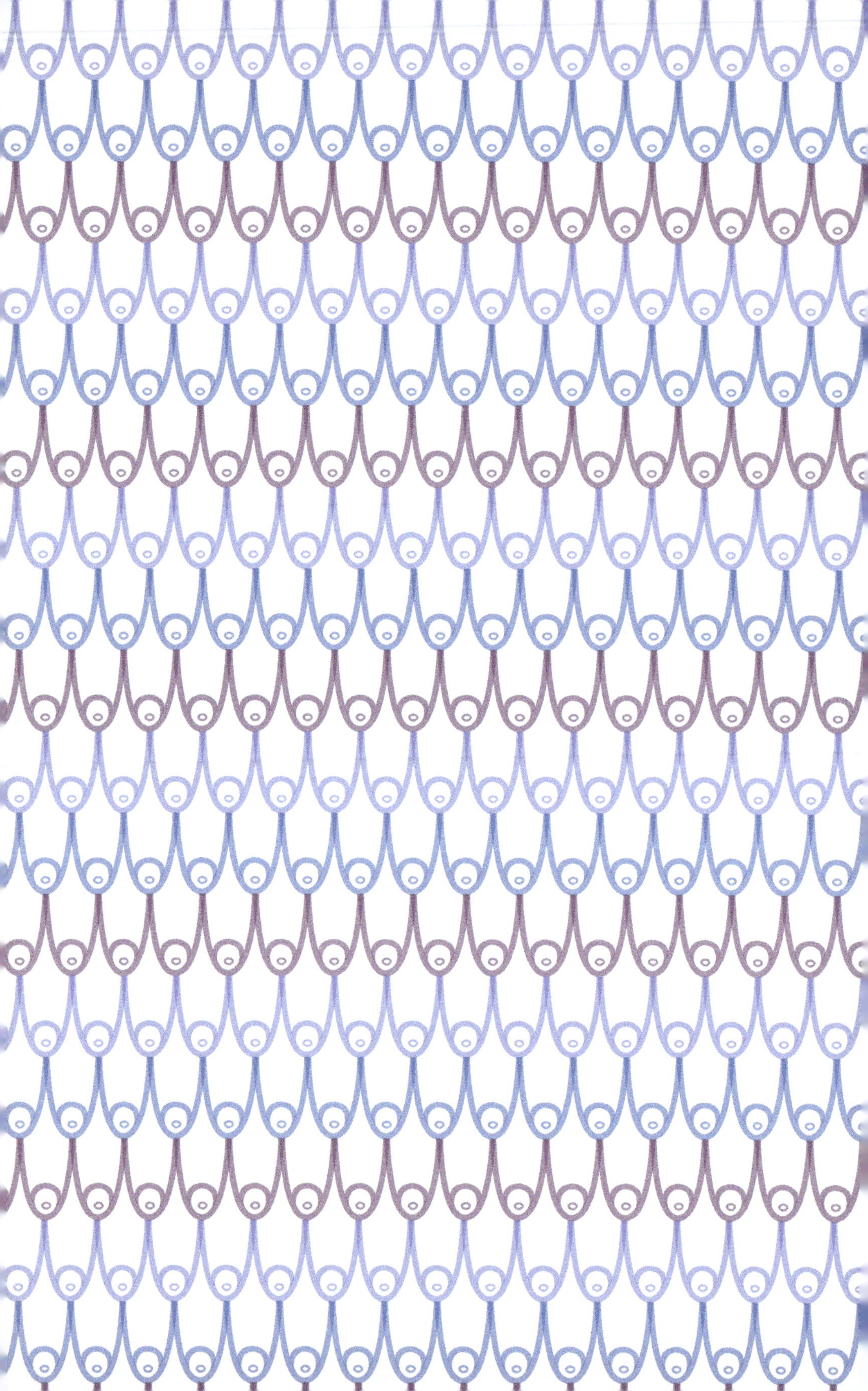

THE MASCULINE ESSENCE

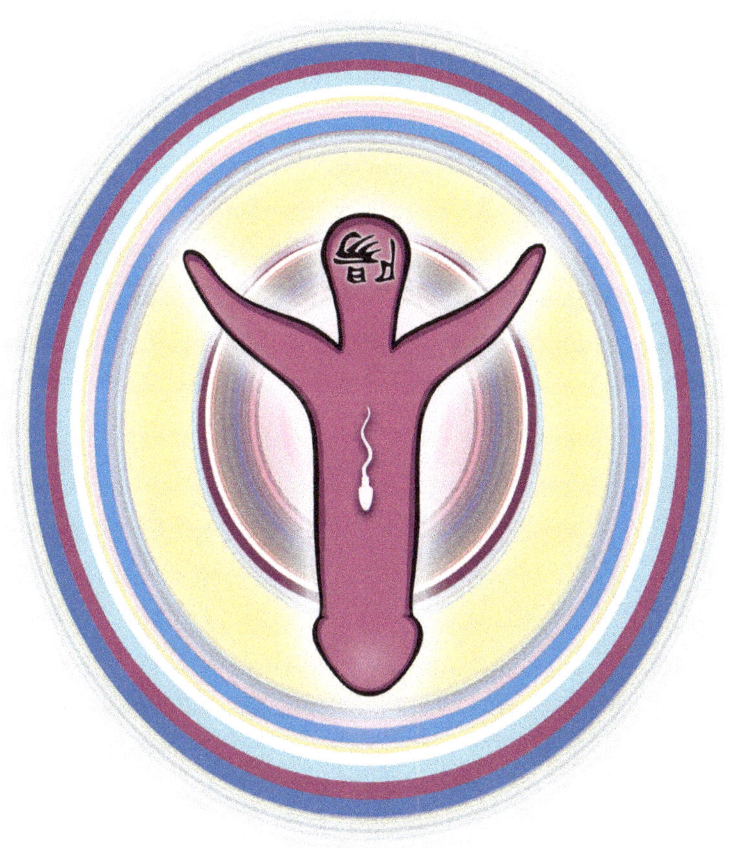

Masculine and feminine

Your gender is determined by whether you have a male or female body, while masculine and feminine energy relate to different states. They are not just concepts but real variants of properties, energy expressions and qualities within us. They are examples of different opposing pairs of our existence. The point here is not that you should be in a particular way or in a particular form, but rather encourages you to explore how you want to express and manage the qualities in your unique way.

The advantage of describing our being from yin and yang is that it helps us see how we can create greater balance in our life and consciously identify which areas we need to develop. For example, how is your balance between activity and rest? Do you need to be more responsive and receptive? Why in that case? How does your balance between thought and feeling look? Regardless of gender, or sexual orientation, the different expressions of yin and yang play different roles on different occasions. Tao encourages all of us to learn from yin and yang how we can create harmony both inside and outside. It involves embracing and exploring both sides and not identifying only with one or the other.

The man's yang nature

As a man, you are born in a man's body and have a male perspective and approach to the outside world. While masculine consciousness includes both yin and yang, most men will live life based on yang principles and derive and communicate primarily from logical thinking and with an aim at the known world. Men start from yang and then learn more of yin while women do the opposite.

If you are a man, your body and your consciousness are expressions of your male potential. The word potential derives from "potent" and means "your capacity, your inherent power and your inner abilities". Perhaps you are aware of them, maybe not. Perhaps you have never thought about exploring your intrinsic powers. A man in balance with his nature has unlimited access to his masculine essence. Essence means what makes someone or something what he or she is, an extract which contains the essentials.

To deepen your understanding you need to explore your yang nature. Yang can be described by words as active, impregnating, awareness, freedom, presence, purpose, expansion, protection, order, delivery, growth, hard, sexy, technical, rational, doing. It is valuable to appreciate these qualities and investigate what the masculine characteristics stand for for you. These qualities are not something you need to look for, but are something that are already inside of you. All you have to do is open yourself up to and receive this endless source of power. It may be easy to feel the essence of yang in different activities with other men, but it can be harder to describe with words. All of these values and qualities are unique and it's about discovering what they mean to you. No one can tell you how to become a "man" since every man is unique. This exploration is a journey you need to do yourself, a journey where you base yourself in your essence and unique combination of abilities.

Your body and your consciousness are expressions of your male potential. The word potential derives from potent and means "your capacity, your inherent power and your inner abilities".

Most of the time, the imprinting of religious dogmas and stereotypical gender roles and body ideals, not least in the media, and our personal history have not favored a free approach to our bodies, our gender, and our inherent naturalness. Traditionally, men were family providers and protected the family and women took care of the children and adorned the homes. These designs are still deeply rooted in us, while modern society has put many new demands on us. In today's western society, the role of the man has become more and more unclear. Being a family provider or successful business person, while baking sourdough and caring for the children, is a challenging combination. The expectations on men to be both strong and sensitive, to look out for yourself while being equal is also not easy to live up to. Some men react by becoming more macho, who exaggerate their masculinity and may even be violent. Others become evasive, which may mean that they completely lose their direction. It is in such situations that we develop imbalances and confusion within us. The changes in gender roles have not been matched by wisdom and guidance in how men can be authentic in their male power. In addition the lack of social acceptance in the male world to explore emotional depths has left many men uninitiated, lost and lonely in their attempt to rediscover new roles on their own. Many men also feel unfairly accused of being the reason for the violent state of the world.

At the same time, women have become more independent and have taken over more "male roles". Women have learned and acquired their yang qualities. Women have fought for and taken on new arenas, more than men, and are usually well educated and can support themselves. Today, 2/3 of university graduates in Sweden are women and surveys say that within ten to fifteen years women will own 60% of the country's financial assets. It is generally both easier and faster for women to adapt. Nevertheless, it is in many ways the masculine power, focusing on the external, that remains the dominant force in society. The outwardly-directed masculine power has dominated for a long time at the expense of the feminine inward-directed force. Imbalances have been created both inside and outside, for both men and women, and in society. And if the distances between us and our nature, between man and woman, between head and heart, between the inner and the outer continue to grow, then we all eventually take damage from the imbalance.

The only way out is in

You need to go inwards to explore your yang nature and masculine essence. In order to do that, you have to stop, take a break and look beyond your inner dialogue. If you cultivate stillness and listen to the silence you will find an inner "mysterious void". This is where you will find your essence, not by searching the outside or comparing yourself to others. This is where you will build your true self-esteem and strength. Based on this inner strength, you can meet the feminine and maintain your yang nature. Freedom means being open to being yourself and being receptive to who you really are.

On the question of what the biggest mistake a man can make, Andrew Fretwell, Wuji gong teacher answers this:

The biggest mistake is that men tend to seek solutions outside of themselves. They are like horses running really fast with blinders on their eyes. Then they suddenly realize that 'This does not work, this is a mistake and is not what I wanted'. If I had a magic wand, I would like to start early to educate young boys at school and help them understand what is really important to them. Finding out what is truly valuable and meaningful has been the key for me.

One of the Nobel prize winners in chemistry said that moments of silence were a factor of his success. He was described as a very creative and happy man. On the question of the secret of his success he answered: "my persistence and my breaks". Every day he locked himself in a room in silence and no one could disturb him. He also said that he welcomed what seemed like "bad" ideas.

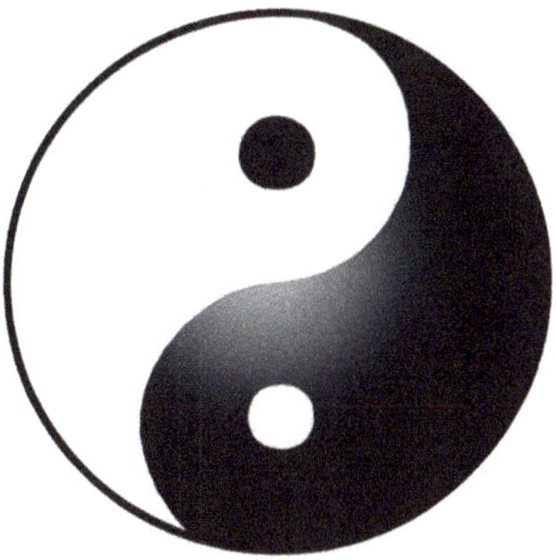

The Taoist philosophy describes yang as strong in the external and weak in the internal. Yin is strong in the inner and weak in the outer. The image of yin and yang shows this clearly with the black (yin) point in the white (yang) field and the white spot in the black field. Yang needs yin to be perfect and vice versa.

The man needs yin

It may seem paradoxical that a man needs to be receptive and susceptible to get to know his masculine essence. He has to turn inwards and contact the feminine, the unknown and the mysterious and not only rely on the obvious and logical. One of the most important tasks a man has is to anchor his feminine pole. In order to become creative, he needs to visit the feminine and explore the unknown and mysterious. The unconscious and undiscovered is unknown until it comes to light and becomes known. It can be anything from disowned feelings and disguised memories to discovering undiscovered abilities, learning new things and exploring new arenas in life.

That exploration also means listening to ideas and thoughts that you don't believe in at the moment. A "besserwisser", one who already knows everything, is the ultimate opposite of a man in contact with his yin side. One wise man has said, "Only a fool is so ignorant that he fakes to know in face of the unknown".

A myth describes the man's journey towards embracing yin, and in turn yang: *The man is likened to the sun and the woman is likened to the earth. In order for a man to become the sun, he has to go out alone in the woods to meet himself. He has to face his fear, his vulnerability and despair. In his helplessness he gives up and then learns to receive the sun. In his enlightenment he becomes receptive and can therefore let in and receive the light. Then he goes back strengthened, knowing he can not understand and solve everything with his head, but needs to open up for a deeper knowledge. True wisdom comes from within and from meeting oneself and the unknown. He then becomes receptive to his creativity and the awareness of, and access to, fruitful, creational power.*

Being only receptive leads to passivity. Only being active becomes a meaningless action. When in contact with both yin and yang, you become receptive to your inherent creative power. You will be responsive to your yin sides without losing the connection to your masculine power. An exercise that strengthens your yin is testicle breathing (see p. 120), where you cultivate your receptivity while you strengthen yang and awaken your power of creation and action.

Man's purpose

According to Tao and many other traditions, the masculine, or yang aspect, manifests thoughts and ideas into the world. Yang qualities are linked with awareness, creational power and intent. For a man, it is extra important to realize purpose in life and to finding valuable goals and meaning. Activity that is not fertilized with meaning is meaningless.

Andrew Fretwell describes:

As I understand, it's important for women to get to know yin, the feminine qualities, in order to develop and absorb yang. And vice versa, men need to get to know their yang qualities to be able to develop and absorb yin. For a man, this means to discover, among other things, what brings him the most joy in life. The more he moves towards his happiness, passion and meaning, the more he moves towards his yang pole. When he finds the content and the connection to his deepest meaning in life there comes a deep relaxation. To accomplish this he needs to go deep into himself, to his yin side, and discover what really lights him up. What makes life really juicy? What makes the soul dance? How do I cultivate my heart's longing for meaning and happiness? Women in turn need to cultivate deep love.

The crux is that in order to really succeed, a man needs to let go of the known and have the courage to explore the unknown. Perhaps this is what adventurous men seek. To stand on the edge and look into the abyss and choose to curiously explore it despite fear. You will then become alert and aware of both what is happening on the outside and what is happening on the inside, in your inner world. The key to success is then to combine the magic of creativity with the knowledge that you already know.

It is important to find out what matters to you in life. It gives a clear direction and an opportunity to realize yourself and share your unique gift with the world. You don't have to save the world. It can be anything from becoming a good dad or a skilled craftsman to expressing feelings and being loving. On page 142 is a small ceremony to guide you towards your purpose.

Powerplay

Sometimes we play different power games to win each other's favor. A man who hasn't acquired self-esteem from his yang nature may play the role of the macho man who knows everything. But deep down, he feels insufficient and insecure. Nevertheless, he uses his sexual power and "just goes for it". Perhaps he chooses to have sex because he is frustrated and wants to "empty" himself. Or he thinks that is what is expected of him, or thinks it's a shame to miss the opportunity. But he does not do it with soul and heart. This behavior gives rise to emptiness and disappointment, it creates feelings of irritation or sudden disinterest. This in turn causes a man to withdraw and separate himself from his lover to feel better, leading to confusion and a desire to condemn or diminish himself and her. The separation comes with a false sense of justification and is one of the reasons why many men feel misunderstood. By not feeling in depth, men deny their nature. By not absorbing and embracing yin as they separate from the feminine and struggle within themselves resulting in a war on two fronts, outside and within.

The same applies to women when they try to "free themselves" from men. Our relationships reflect us. Recurring themes in relationships often have their foundation in our family constellations from childhood or inherited patterns from generations back. A common theme is based on our various positive and negative poles. A woman's positive pole is in her heart. This means that women focus more on emotions and communication. A man's positive pole is in the genitals and is therefore more focused on sex. If he is emotionally unbalanced, he has a tendency to "just go for it" and then run away after the sexual interaction, as he experiences women as emotionally demanding. Several men have confirmed that they run away when they think a woman is demanding and because it is scary to get tied up. The more men pull away, the more women chase them for confirmation. And contrarily, a woman runs away when the man just wants sex, and therefore he continues to chase his prey. After a sexual encounter, a man usually has an easier time to just move on, while a woman wants to understand and analyze what happened. Men run because they are afraid to hurt. Women defend men through love and understanding. That way we "take care of each other". These behaviors and attitudes do not enhance relationships. When the poles are imbalanced, we create addictions. We look for in each other for things that we do not have access to in ourselves. A man who unilaterally searches for ejaculation and orgasm, without the ability of emotional connection, is as half and incomplete as a woman seeking to be close without the ability of sexual dedication.

Of course, there are many ways to create imbalances between yang and yin, men and women, masculine and feminine. The examples above that many men distance themselves from both their feelings and the feminine is a generalization. There are men who do the opposite, which causes them to drain their energy through a surplus of yin. They become too adaptable, fail in their decision-making capacity and lose their own purpose. They are constantly seeking confirmation from women, perhaps they even think that too "male" men are a little unpleasant. Today, it is also not uncommon that women have a well-developed yang side and grab for themselves without any demands on emotional involvement. The variations are many.

> *A man who unilaterally searches for ejaculation and orgasm, without the ability of emotional connection, is as half and incomplete as a woman seeking to be close without the ability of sexual dedication.*

This is something for you to explore. Why not go live and experiment a little? Dare to throw yourself into the unknown and explore new ways to be. Initially, it can arouse resistance and create a feeling of insecurity. Good practice may be to look at a kind of art you do not know, listen to music you usually don't listen to, or to learn something completely new. In this way you will learn that there are many areas you neither know or understand. What will be the difference in your approach compared to old habitual situations? Which feels most creative, playful and attractive? In what new ways do you want to meet and curiously explore the feminine? Or a new partner? With what attitude? What gives you energy, excitement, happiness and joy?

Man is activity, woman is stillness

Tao says that the man is active in his essence and therefore searches for silence, magic and the unknown. The woman is silent in her essence and therefore seeks development, movement and the known. A friend and colleague, Eric, 45, described this interaction between feminine and masculine energy with dance as metaphor: *In tango the movements are controlled by the music, but within that frame it is free. The interaction between the man and the woman is based on mutual receptivity. The woman guides by sensing and showing the way. The man leads by listening where the energy goes. At the same time as he leads, he lets himself be guided. The woman, in turn, is willing to be led, while being responsive and inviting to the movement.*

Eric finds that it happens quite often that women do not let themselves be led, but they'd rather want to control, and then it becomes "this is how it's done" and not free anymore. It may also happen that the woman is a victim, "dance me" and the man begins to control instead of leading. Then he is scolded for it. When the man wants too much in the dance (the love making), it is good if the woman can guide and keep the presence in the meeting.

If both of them stopped listening to each other, and the steps in the dance were purely technical, the dance would not be good. It becomes a dance without feeling, respect and togetherness. It is about coming from the essence, intuition and evolvement together in the state of being and to be open and prepared for different and new experiences. When a couple dances with the heart, one can not see who leads or who follows, they have become one with the dance!

Imbalanced interplay

A common dilemma is the man who finds that his wife has a great need for control and confirmation. She may be a strong woman with many of her own problems, but who is not in touch with her own feelings. Instead, she requires the man to conform to her emotional needs. She is fully occupied with herself and unaware of the needs of her husband. The man may work and struggle, but he will feel like he is scolded for it, and he then feels useless. He gets angry and irritated and withdraws and maybe starts to work more. Then he has no ability to see and confirm his wife. The woman, in turn, feels unhappy and also starts feeling useless. If the woman does not feel seen, she begins to complain. Many men find that their women complain about them working too much. He gets angry because she doesn't support him in his work. At the same time he doesn't realize that the job may be eating him, taking all his power, destroying his marriage, health and his life. Both are dissatisfied.

Many men also find that their woman not only wants to refurbish the living room, but also wants to change him. This is perceived negatively and can in the worst case cause him to feel unappreciated. Sometimes, however, it may be appropriate for a man to listen to his wife when she expresses dissatisfaction. Many men are surprised when their wives "suddenly" want to separate. They have not wanted to, or been unable to see that the relationship needed to be deepened or changed, wondering what has happened and feel like they don't "recognize" their partner.

Another common way to misunderstand each other is based on our different needs when getting home from work. Needing to unwind from the stresses of the day, the man often wants to withdraw, which the woman perceives as a rejection. The woman, in turn, wants to talk about the day and the man feels invaded.

The man needs to feel appreciated and get recognition for what he does. He finds satisfaction in finding solutions to problems and reaching goals. Because the woman in many ways is a mystery to herself, she has to be seen and confirmed for who she is. Many times, it only requires a pair of alert ears and full attention and presence from someone. She doesn't need solutions, just someone who listens. The unknown is a mystery and will remain as such.

A woman in her career, as well as a mother, tends to embrace her "masculine side". The yang side of her is also triggered by an indecisive and uncertain man who leaves responsibility and decision to the woman in the family. Then she soon has no man, but a little boy and she is no wife, but a mother. This doesn't promote the relationship, sex life or personal development. Instead, it risks creating major problems. The parties eventually end up tire of each other, become condemning and withdrawn, unfaithful or even aggressive. This situation is common all over the world and described in the book "The Toltec Teachings", by the author Theun Mares who depict this as a major problem, between men and women.

Men's fear of intimacy and closeness is rooted deep in mankind, and it can certainly apply to women too. According to a psychological theory, it is the result of an ongoing process of liberation of a little boy striving to distance himself from the mother to become an independent individual. Intimacy and closeness become a threat also against the independence of the grown man. They form a kind of "love hate relationship" that forces away empathy and love. A structure that makes it difficult for some men to see how, for example, porn violates people and trivializes sexuality. Real feelings, on the contrary, remove the distance needed for unhealthy consumption of porn.

These are some examples of imbalanced interplay between different people that nobody really needs to take personally. Whether the behavior originates in our biology or culture, they are often unconscious and do not have much to do with the current partner. The same situations will be played out even if the partner is replaced, until the pattern is broken and you see that you are the cause of your dissatisfaction. How do you think and act? How happy are you in your relationship? How can you support yourself and your partner so that you become more aware and can communicate and handle your needs in a better way? It can be a good idea to sit down every now and then and share with each other what your needs are, what you want, as well as what you want to give.

In many cases, men need to be more masculine and determined, and women need to be better at affirming their feminine and receptive sides, especially in our close relationships. Moreover, in order for an attraction between men and women to occur, a certain polarization is required. If we become more conscious, we can understand how these poles, the masculine and the feminine interact, and it is a development that goes hand in hand with your own self-acceptance and inner balance between yin and yang. A genius is one who can hold opposites. The Taoist approach to the man's yang nature contains insights and wisdom that are well worth exploring.

Man's liberation

Women's liberation has been highlighted and discussed in various forms for many years. But what does the man's liberation look like? Why doesn't interest in male development seem to be the same? Here's an attempt to shed light on some questions. Men are in a position of power, and women subordinate. The gender hierarchies live through informal, often unconscious, thought patterns. Periodically, the "old" image of male sexuality pops up. When the media highlights men's violence against women, it's almost always the victim who is discussed and not the perpetrator. We rarely bring up the possibility of addressing the problem itself, finding the background of the behavior and helping the men who commit abuse to change. If we don't redirect focus from the victim, then how can it change over time? Instead, one continues to describe the man as a more or less unaware creature with an uncontrollable drive that makes him recklessly go after what he craves. How can man rid himself of his sexual buoy and his insensitive prison? What new ideas and images of the "new" man's sexuality do you want to be a part of and create?

Women have struggled to adapt to the ups and downs of our economically fluctuating society. They have, for better and for worse, adopted male attributes. Hanna Rosin in her book "The End of Men" shows in her analysis of cultural, economic and sexual changes in power dynamics how men are being caught up to and overtaken by women in field after field. Boys are finding school difficult and men begin to fall behind both in terms of education and work, making their role in society erratic and unreliable.

So where is male liberation? How can men help each other to develop the uniquely male expression of power and beauty? How can men and women together create a successful partnership between the sexes with a balance between yin and yang? Hopefully, we will continue our existence on this planet, so we need to find sustainable solutions, and enterprising and receptive people who can work together, listen and anticipate and make informed decisions for the generations to come.

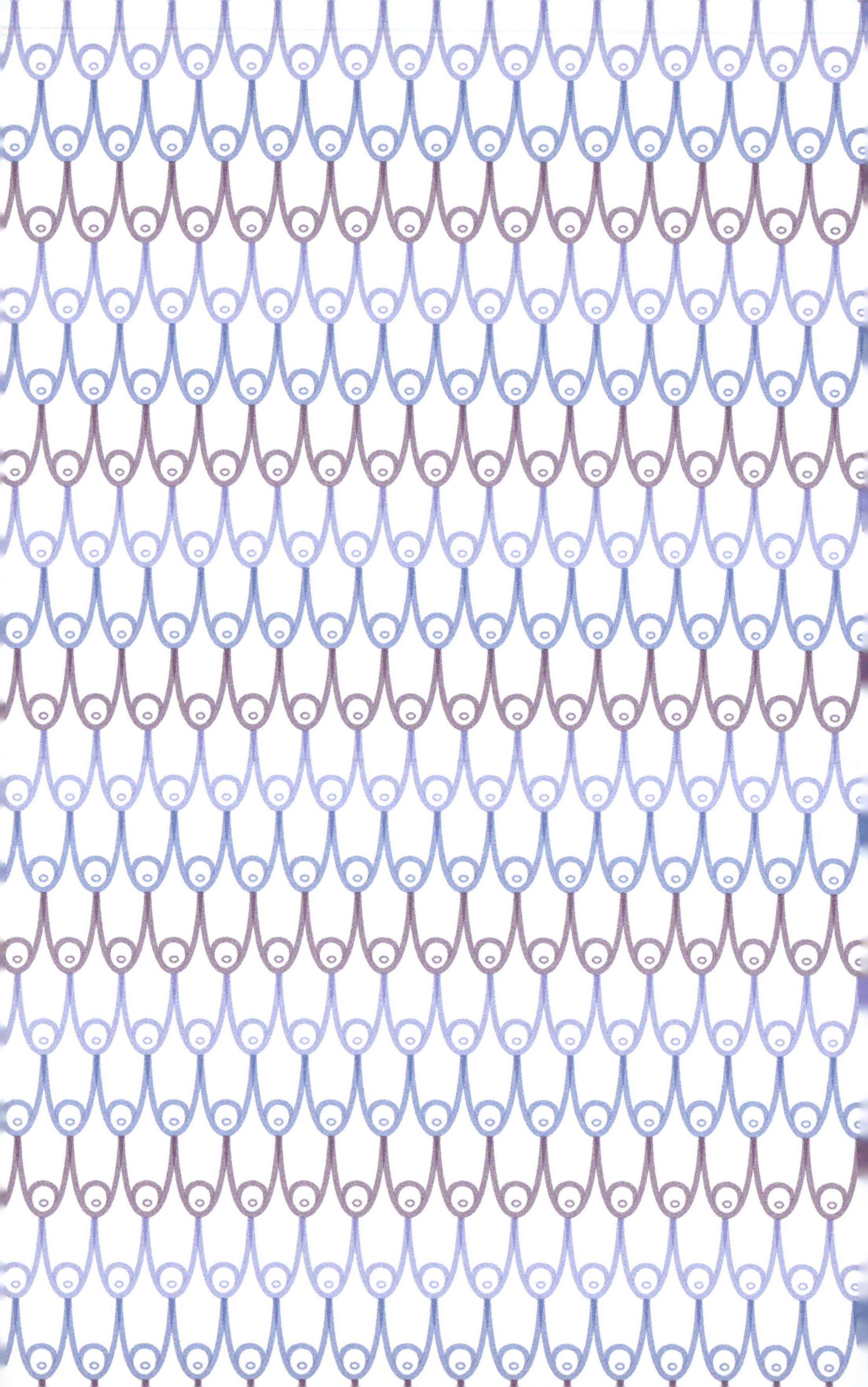

THE PATH
OF LIFE

Life's natural cycles

Nature and life are constantly changing and going through different events. The seasons clearly show how life, death, transformation and regeneration interact. In the universe, everything has its own rhythm, follows its own cycle and is governed by its universal law. The woman has her natural cycle of menstruation in accordance with the moon. There are men who feel that, like water on the planet, they are also affected by the movements of the moon. One man talked about becoming melancholic at every full moon (which he found out with great surprise). To him, it is a clear and regular signal that it is time for reflection and turning his eyes inward. He is used to not setting up important meetings at that time. Another finds that he often becomes more emotional and has difficulty sleeping around the full moon. A third says he has his "male period". You can "sneak" up on yourself and see if you have any recurring themes in your life that follow a special rhythm or cycle.

> *You can't change the life cycle, just face it with respect and humility. You can choose to gain more knowledge and to have a curious new attitude.*

Men also have their own life cycles with different stages - from childhood and teens to a young fertile man on his way out into life. Then come the adult years along with work, career, paternity and family. After that, the full grown, experienced man appears, then comes the old age, which hopefully ends with the wise grandfather. According to Chinese medicine, every age has its events. If you as a teenager have the same lifestyle as an adult man or if an old man lives as a youth, it creates imbalance because our needs and conditions are different in different ages. For example, hormone systems and muscle systems change with age.

Previously, there were transitional rituals for the different stages of development so that people could more easily adapt and continue to develop. You can't change the cycle of life, just face it with respect and humility. You can choose to gain more knowledge, have a curious attitude and follow the changes.

Sexual maturity

The most obvious change in man's life occurs in the teens when the sex hormones in the body completely explode and all bodily and mental changes begin. Puberty clearly shows the effects the hormone testosterone has. The muscles grow, the puberty voice change begins, the beard grows, the testicles grow and the sex drive increases. From the first ejaculation in pre-puberty, the man is considered to be sexually mature. The man is then fertile with the opportunity to create children for the rest of his life. The newly awoken sex hormones act as an invigorating agent and enhance performance, fertility and libido.

Young man

Growing up as a young man today and integrating sexuality, sensuality, body and feelings is not easy. It belongs to puberty to be self-centered and wondering who you are. The changes are drastic and many worry about whether they are ok. It can be anything from the size of the penis and how the scrotum is hanging to the amount and color of the sperm. These are worries that sometimes accompany someone throughout their entire life.

It is of course good that a young man is exploring his sexuality, but to know where the boundaries are is more difficult. When do I risk going too far, how can I feel safe, what do I really want? Sweden has had compulsory sexual education in school since the 1950s and that is good. Nevertheless, it can be difficult for young people to get authentic answers to their questions about sexuality from an adult. Many adults themselves have tensions around sexuality. The advice we get will then be general and may perhaps be examples of what we should not do, like; do not get someone pregnant or, think about sexually transmitted diseases before you have sex. Sometimes teaching also becomes too technical and mechanical. Such as in "this is how it works, penis in and out of a vagina, and use a condom". Perhaps there is some truth in Sister Sofi's words from the book Kroppens Teologi, "Theology of the Body" where she writes: *we talk about sex as if sexuality was a leisure activity among many others; use a life jacket when you ride a boat, helmet when you ride a bike, and a condom when you have sex.* Have we de-personified sexuality? Has love making completely lost its deeper meaning? In combination with today's world of the internet, the technical and distancing sex becomes even more apparent. What's missing is the feeling and the magic. How many young men get to learn that sex is something natural, sacred and beautiful? That they are a person with heart and dreams to be taken seriously? That it's normal to be afraid, insecure and sensitive to criticism? Sexual frustration is the cause of many problems, ranging from poor self-esteem and depression to abuse and violence. Sexual maturity means having a positive comprehension about ones body, genitals, sexuality and trust in our own and the opposite sex.

Contraceptives

Throughout his adult life, the man is fertile and able to impregnate the woman. So far, there are few alternatives to condoms as contraception for men. There have been "contraceptive pills" for men, but since the hormone preparations have failed to meet the safety and efficacy requirements, they are not interesting. An option as a contraceptive for men is sterilization, which is called a vasectomy. Then the tubes of the vas deferens are cut and tied. This prevents the sperm from getting out of the testes. The operation is done with local anesthesia and doesn't take long and the side effects are few. Even if sterilization is to be seen as a permanent procedure, it is possible to once again make a man fertile. Either have the seminal ducts sewn back together, or have them directly connected to the epididymis where sperm mature. The actual production of sperm is continuing throughout life and hormone production is not affected by the procedure. Sperm is only a small part of the ejaculation and therefore you ejaculate other seminal fluids even if you had a vasectomy.

Sperm quality

The biological clock also ticks for men. Sperm count and quality, meaning mobility, shape, volume and concentration, deteriorate with age. However, it has been found that the male reproductive ability has deteriorated radically over the past decades. In the 1940s, an ejaculation consisted of 150 million sperm per ml. and today it is about approx. 15 million per ml. An ejaculation contains 3-5 ml. During the same period, the quality of sperm has fallen by 50% in American men. Researchers in Denmark have seen the same trends. Many couples have trouble getting pregnant, and 7-8% remain biologically childless. In about half of the cases, childlessness is due to the fact that the man has a reduced or in some cases a complete lack of reproductive capacity. Part of the problem arises from the increased chemical stress on our society and endocrine disruptors that leak into our home environment through plastics. Even residues of hormone treatments and birth control pills are flushed into our water and end up in the drinking water. It also seems that the poisons accumulate in our offspring.

Testosterone

The most important male sex hormone is testosterone. The center of production is in the brain, where the hypothalamus controls through the pituitary gland and regulates hormone levels as needed. The testosterone is then formed in the testicles and excreted into the bloodstream. The amount of testosterone in the blood is reported to the brain which, based on that information, corrects the hormone levels. It is the amount of free testosterone in the blood that affects the sperm, seminal vesicles and prostate secretion. In absence of testosterone in the blood, there will be no sperm. When you're excited or happy, the production is stimulated. During stress and anger, it is reduced. Stress hormones always win over sex hormones. Decreased amounts of testosterone can lead to ill-health as well as difficulty getting an erection along with a lack of self-esteem. Erections are important for the man's virility and pride and his identity is often associated with his sexual ability. With the exercises in this book you can prevent stress and promote production of sex hormones, health and potency.

The testosterone decreases

Testosterone levels are at their peak in the 20-30s and they then start to gradually decrease. The testosterone probably begins to decrease by about 1% per year from the 30s and 40s. So the hormone decline in men occurs gradually as compared to the hormone reduction in women taking place more drastically. During this transition, women may suffer from heat strokes, dry mucous membranes and mood swings.

Symptoms of testosterone deficiency are often more diffuse and vary from individual to individual. The three most obvious markers for testosterone deficiency are: no morning erection, difficulty in maintaining the erection, and difficulty in conducting intercourse. Other common symptoms include decreased sex lust, decreased muscle mass, increased abdominal fat, osteoporosis, fatigue and irritation. There are split opinions regarding what it means when your levels of testosterone are too low. The lack of testosterone is not the same as the need for treatment. One should show symptoms as well. Far from everyone shows any symptoms, despite low testosterone levels. Several of the symptoms of testosterone deficiency are similar to, and may therefore be confused with, other conditions such as depression, stress, obesity, diabetes, smoking, alcohol, environmental problems etc. Testosterone levels may also be affected by various medications and conditions. The medical term for testosterone deficiency is hypogonadism.

Andropause

As men grow older, the testosterone content gradually decreases and some men experience a male climacterium. Andrology is Greek and means "the teaching of man" and men's "menopause" is called andropause. It describes a stage in the adult man's life when the production of testosterone decreases. The male andropause "was discovered" already in the late 18th century by Dr. Hooper. He considered it a disease. In 1935, it was possible to produce synthetic testosterone and in the mid 1940s a number of men were treated with noticeable results, though some unwelcome side effects did occur. Only in recent years, at the end of the 1990s, did we begin to talk about the significance of hormones for men. But it is still controversial whether the andropause is a disease that should be treated or if it's a natural process, like the menopause in women. The andropause usually occurs around 50-55 years. One figure that is sometimes mentioned is that about 10% of men experience inconveniences. Another study shows that about 5% of men in their 50s are affected by the symptoms, and those over 70 years old experience up to 50% of the symptoms. You can feel the symptoms without perceiving them as inconvenient.

There are some critical voices to the term andropause. They don't question the existence of the andropause but the emergence of it as a medical term as well as the link to research and drug companies' medicalization of society. A diagnosis leads to more drugs being produced and printed. Others say that the man remains fertile throughout his life, and the testosterone levels fall slowly, and therefore the term andropause is not relevant.

Middle age crisis

Andropause is often kept apart from the middle age crisis some men can end up in. Sometimes they come at the same time. Middle age crisis is seen as a social and psychological process, while the andropause is seen as a biochemical process where hormones affect the life experience. Both of these phenomena would most likely affect each other and any inconvenience could reflect your lifestyle. Your biochemistry is influenced by how you feel and how you live your life and vice versa.

A middle age crisis is associated with a turning point in life that has to do with external circumstances. The children have grown up, the career climb is cleared, the marriage is about to be dissolved or deepened. Old delusions are dissolved while new horizons have not yet taken shape. All of this can create feelings of confusion and uncertainty. It affects your identity and purpose in life. As you age and the testosterone decreases you may feel that your sex drive is going down. One gift is that it becomes natural to slow down. You may want to explore deeper needs for closeness and intimacy as well as new ways to have sex. It's time to stop and orient yourself towards new goals. In the past, different old cultures had transitional rituals for all transitional stages of life. You simply made the final accounts and set aims towards new goals. According to Tao, lack of direction and sense of purpose robs you of your life energy. The male burden of performance and the stress of today's living are also important factors in creating a midlife crisis.

Take time to stop and think about your values every now and then. What is really important to you? How do you want to live for the rest of your life?

We all need to take a break periodically to review our values and ask ourselves if we invest our energy in what is really important to us. How do you want to continue living the rest of your life? On page 142 there is an exercise you can try for greater clarity.

Prostate awareness

It is common that the prostate increases in size with age. Since the prostate is situated around the urethra, an enlarged prostate can block the urine. The first symptoms are often diffuse pain and difficulty peeing. Or you pee often, having to get up in the middle of the night and it stings and hurts.

The correlation between prostate size and severity of symptoms is quite weak, and a significant enlargement doesn't need to cause any inconvenience. The enlargement passes after some time, or remains without causing any trouble. With aging, the bladder may also become weaker and the urination reflex will not work as well, which may have similar symptoms to an enlarged prostate. So in the case of urination, it may be difficult to determine how many of the problems depend on the prostate or a weak bladder. Urinary tract infection also produces similar symptoms, such as urgency, burning and aching pain. Often the symptoms are due to tense muscles in the pelvic floor and not the UTI.

Enlargement of the prostate may not be something that has anything to do with normal ageing, but could be a consequence of something in the western lifestyle. In some cultures, like in China and Japan, having a prostate problem is more rare than in the US and Europe. If a Chinese person moves to the US, he increases the risk of being affected. Age, heritage, lifestyle and where you live in the world are risk factors as well as conditions like abdominal obesity, high blood pressure, high blood sugar and poor blood fats. Hormone imbalances caused by depression, stress and anxiety have also been noted in connection with prostate issues, and even dietary effects, foods rich in saturated fats, trans fat and high calorie.

A sedentary life and lack of exercises play a large factor. Sitting causes constant pressure to the prostate and prevents circulation, which can lead to oxygen deficiency and the occurrence of pain. Excessive bicycling has been shown to have a negative impact on the prostate. In addition to this, for various reasons, the pelvic floor muscles can be constantly tense and affect the situation of the genital area. Cramps in the pelvic floor muscles may be a symptom of both long-term pressure and stress.

Most prostatic enlargements are benign. At the same time prostate cancer is one of the most common forms of cancer in men in the western world. Most people who are affected are over 70 years old. At the age of 80, about 80% of men have small tumors in the prostate, but most of them never know. If you are worried and have severe pain or problems with your pelvic floor or prostate go and see a doctor and do a check up to exclude infection or prostate illness!

The prostate is your "inner heart" and located in the center of your body. Think about it with ease and give your prostate attention, love and appreciation.

Prostatitis and pelvic floor pain

Prostatitis is a collective name for issues in or around the prostate gland and in the male genital area. Prostatitis is described in two forms - acute and chronic. Acute prostatitis is an inflammation which occurs suddenly. It is always caused by bacteria.

The chronic is divided into "chronic bacterial prostatitis" and "chronic pelvic floor syndrome", before called "chronic nonbacterial prostatitis". Chronic bacterial prostatitis means that you have difficulty and pain for a long time. The reason is usually unknown, but can sometimes be due to bacteria.

In case of "chronic pelvic floor syndrome", it is believed to be tense muscles of the pelvic floor and doesn't have anything to do with the prostate. One theory is that the muscles cramp up and create a sort of "headache" in the pelvic area. Inflammation can occur because the muscles of the pelvic floor are constantly tense, just as an over-tight muscle in a shoulder may be irritated and inflamed.

About 90% of those affected by prostatitis have "chronic pelvic floor syndrome" with diffuse pelvic floor pain. About 10% of men suffer from it at some point during life.

Symptoms and treatment:

- Chronic pelvic floor syndrome: diffuse pain in the pelvic floor and back, heavy feeling in the lower abdominal area, shooting pain and sore genitals, pain when ejaculating, weaker erection, urinary issues, needing to go to the toilet more often, weaker stream, inefficient emptying, after drops of urine, symptoms and pain varies in intensity and may relapse, or cease. Ways to go to treat the condition is to release the tension and understand how it arises. Treatment can include physical work on the pelvic floor muscles, awareness exercises, relaxation, mindfulness and stress reduction.

- Acute prostatitis: abdominal pain and urination issues, sore and aching prostate, sometimes high fever. If you get a fever, consult a doctor immediately. In case of acute conditions, treatment with antibiotics usually has a good effect

- Chronic bacterial prostatitis: the symptoms and pain vary in intensity, acute inflammation can develop. Tend to pass by themselves. If the symptoms are not due to bacteria or inflammation, antibiotics don't help.

Physical therapy of the pelvic floor is recommended both in alternative and conventional health care. Even prostate massage was previously used in medical care. Further into this book you will learn both pelvic floor training and beneficial prostate massage that helps keep the prostate healthy, agile and potent. Squeezing exercises, genital massages and healthy sexual activity can promote a more healthy pelvic floor. The prostate is your "inner heart" and located in the center of your body. Think about it with ease and give your prostate attention, love and appreciation.

Pelvic diaphragm from above

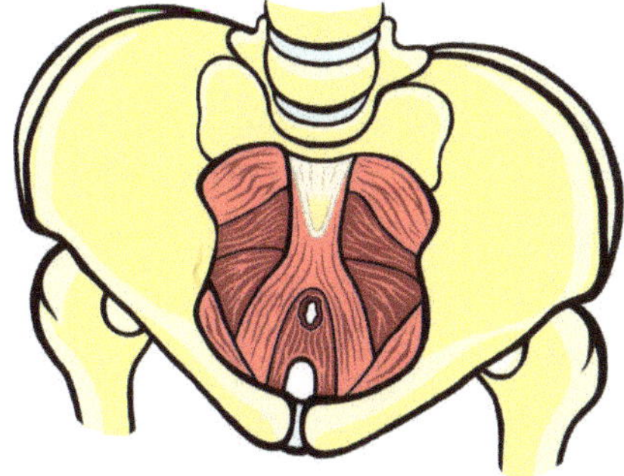

The pelvic floor supports your prostate and sexual health.

Male incontinence

Male incontinence is more common than most think and affects approx 10-20 % of the population and increases with age. A problem that is not much spoken about and not many seek help for. Three types of incontinence are seen. Stress incontinence is caused when an increase in abdominal pressure happens, such as laughing, coughing and sneezing. Things that may help causing this can be bad posture, dysfunctional pelvic floor, lack of physical training and obesity. Urge incontinence is a sudden and strong need to go to pee and is sometimes caused by an enlarged prostate pressing on the bladder. Overflow incontinence means difficulty to hold pee in and can also be caused by an enlarged prostate or a bladder that is too stretched out.

Tense pelvic muscles can prevent the urine from being emptied properly when peeing or cause the prostate to empty poorly during ejaculation, which may cause an obtuse discomfort in the lower abdomen as a consequence. Both the prostate and the muscles are centrally located and several nerves pass by, so a swollen prostate or tense muscles could cause many different inconveniences. The exercises in this book will support the function of the muscles in the pelvic floor and help prevent incontinence.

Abdominal fat

Do you belong to those who suddenly walk around with an extra big stomach? You're not alone. Unfortunately, this is a type of obesity that can be risky and linked to both prostatitis and several of our common lifestyle diseases such as hypertension, diabetes and sleep apnea. If you are over about 39 inches in circumference by the navel, you are in the risk zone. The easiest way to do something about this is to review your diet, especially reducing unhealthy fats and carbohydrates and reducing portions. And exercise more. Reduced muscle mass leads to reduced metabolism. Stress affects the entire hormone system and is an underestimated reason for obesity.

Aging and Tao

A term that often occurs in the Taoist philosophy is "immortality". Its meaning is widely discussed. Some mean literal immortality where the body through techniques can be preserved as long as the practitioner wants. Another interpretation is that the soul, or consciousness, remains intact even after the end of life. Tao and several other thought traditions describe the moment of death as the most important in life and that life is a preparation for the last breath. A Taoist saying is: "You never die because you were never born, you've only forgotten who you are". For thousands of years, Tao has refined natural and practical methods for developing human nature and prolonging life. If we are in good health, we can live well over a hundred years. The foundation for a good life is a balance of the "three treasures of life energy". These uplifting Taoist Qigong exercises do not stop aging, but help you keep your vitality alive even in your older days. They are no "miracle cure" but require time, dedication and regularity, but offer a lot of enjoyment along the way. Tao also encourage us to explore our "immortality" and who we truly are. The exercises support you to embody your spirituality and awaken your inner light. Every human soul is unique but, also from the same great consciousness.

> *For thousands of years, Tao has refined natural and practical methods for developing human nature and prolonging life.*

Sex and health

Today, it's not just Tao that connects sex and health. There has been a lot of studies on how sexuality affects our well-being. They have shown that enriching your sex life promotes your immune systems, strengthens the heart and raises the general experience of a good life. A reasonable amount of sex balances the hormone system and lowers cholesterol and blood pressure. The orgasm is an internal phenomenon that balances the biochemistry and hormones of the body.

Create time for self-reflection

The Taoists thus describe our sexual energy, our orgasmic flows and the masculine essence as an elixir of youth. They created exercises to cultivate life energy. Even if you don't have a partner or a relationship with an active sex life, it's very worthwhile to still train your libido. Creating space for self-reflection is fundamental as well. My hope is that the exercises in this book will help you on your way to be readily prepared to meet life in a more balanced way. Although the world is not always a peaceful place, there is the opportunity to create harmony in your relationship with yourself and thus with your surroundings. Remember that no one can take away your power and you can't take it back either. But you can learn to feel that it has never been lost, but has always been there.

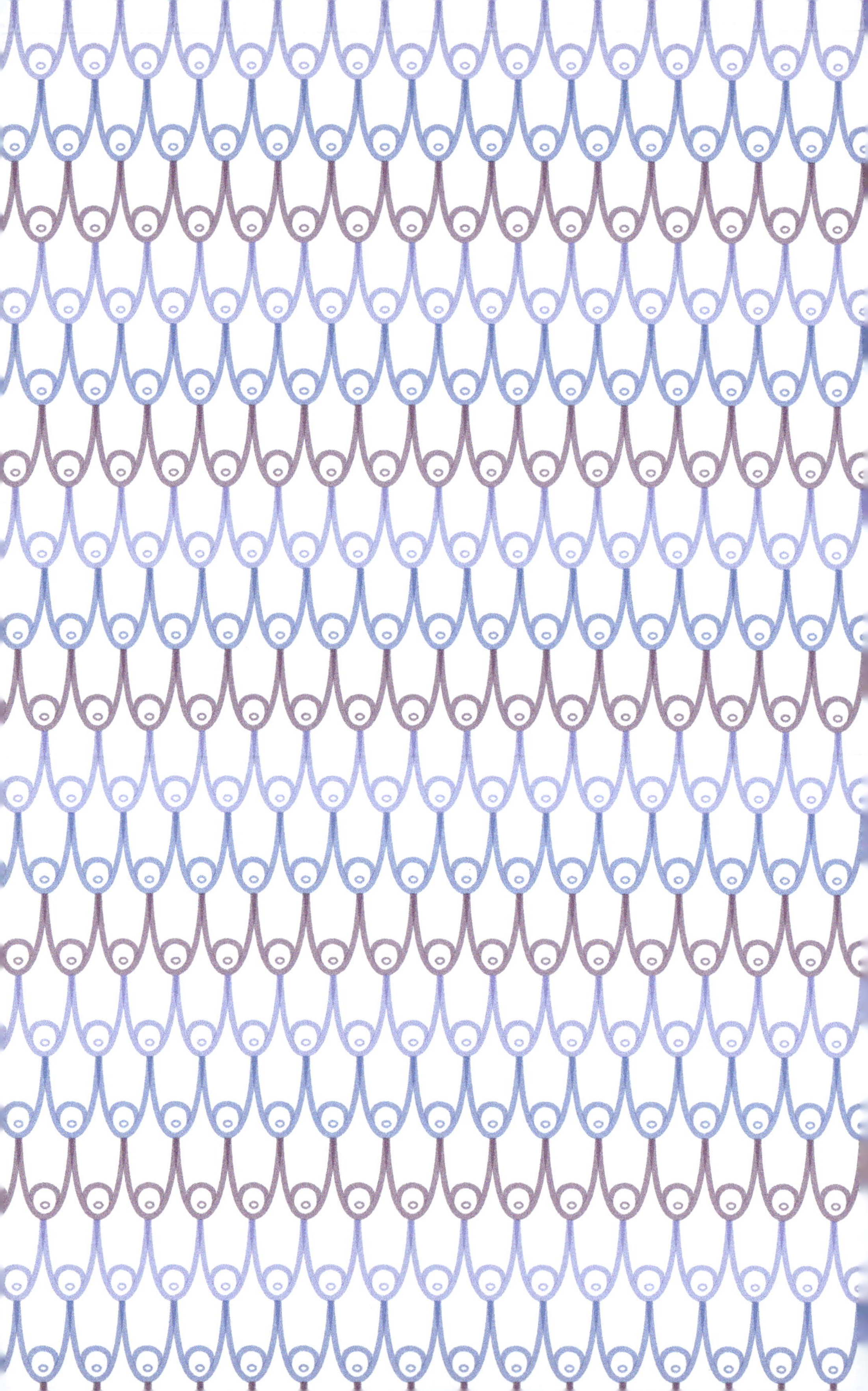

EXERCISES

Before the exercises

Several of the exercises that follow are guided meditations where you move your attention around the body with the power of thought. You use your awareness to guide the energy. Have a clear focus, an open mind and a curious attitude during your exploration. Keep in mind that when you focus inward you can use the breath to get in touch with different body parts. As a rule, you breathe in and out through your nose. Your inner eyes help you to see and your inner ears help you to listen to your inner world. You can rely on your presence and your intentions to make a difference. All exercises are designed to create or restore a natural flow.

Prior to each exercise I recommend preparatory exercises and sometimes also finishing exercises. The exercises build on each other to some extent, but all can be done individually. I do, however, always recommend starting with basic positions (exercise 1) to create a supportive posture. Finish with collecting the Qi you've generated (exercise 3), in order for the vital life force energy to be preserved.

Different reactions

In the beginning you may feel tired when you concentrate for a long time. But that feeling usually passes and is a response to resistance or energy that comes into motion, as well as the habit of associating relaxation with sleep. You may also feel tingling, vibrating or prickly sensations when you release tension. Other reactions may be burps and yawning. If you get dizzy then open your eyes and focus on your breathing and on your feet. Take your time and respect your limitations.

Emotional reaction

Sometimes memories with related emotions and history unravel. The recommendation is to not try to avoid the emotion or resist it, but take a neutral, observing and accepting attitude towards it. Thoughts and feelings come and flow constantly, and they belong to your life energy, no matter what form they are taking at the moment. Through these exercises, and through your presence, your unprocessed emotions can be transformed and restored to life-giving power.

NOTE!

If you are of ill health, whether mental or physical, or feel unsure if an exercise is good for you, contact your doctor, another professional contact or speak with an experienced Qigong instructor.

Basic positions

Here's a guide to finding a good foundation, a good starting point within yourself, for both sitting and standing exercises. Your posture affects both your breathing and Qi flow. To have a special place or room where you do the exercises is also recommended.

Guide exercise 1:

Time: 5 min, sitting or standing

Purpose: Correct your posture ❤ Turn your attention inward ❤ Connection to heaven and earth

Standing basic position:

Stand with parallel feet, approximately hip width apart and with your toes straight ahead. Softly bend your ankles, knees and hips and relax your groin. Pull your tailbone slightly in between your legs so that the lower back is smooth and becomes straight. Let your arms hang along the sides and have an open feeling in your chest. Guide your sternum slightly forward and upward, to get your shoulders into place. Your chin is slightly pulled in to have your neck become an extension of the spine. Notice where the center of gravity is in your footpads and swing back and forth, and from side to side to find equilibrium.

Sitting basic position:

Sit far out on the chair, on your sit bones with your feet firm on the ground. Alternatively you can sit on the floor in meditation position with your legs crossed. The back is erect and straight. Have an open feeling in your chest. Guide your sternum slightly forward and upward to get your shoulders into place. Your chin is slightly pulled in to have your neck become an extension of the spine. Place your hands in each other, right hand in left, slightly below the navel.

Continuation for both standing and sitting:

Then close your eyes (alternatively fix your eyes at a point on the ground) and turn your focus inwards. Relax in your mind and rest into yourself. Be aware of your breathing and take a few deep breaths. Guide your breath to your lower belly and let your mind sink down to your center in Dan Tian, below and behind the navel. Let the mind rest in your breath. Put the tip of your tongue on the palate, slightly behind your teeth, where the gum becomes a bit softer, teeth apart and relaxed jaw. Push upwards 3 times. Keeping the tongue there through all exercises is recommended.

Move your attention down to your tailbone. Then move your attention up the spine, vertebra after vertebra, up to the neck and the base of the skull and lengthen your spine from within. Feel the ascending, upright force. The one who wants to be awake and alert. Be aware of and touch the space or the sky above you. Then receive the descending force, the relaxation and gravitational pull. Relax your face, around your eyes, behind your eyes and in your jaw. Shoulders and chest relax. The back, abdomen and legs relax. Then feel your feet and touch the ground and earth below.

Now you are in a good position to continue with any other exercise.

Physical warm-up exercises

Here are some warm-up exercises that will help you loosen up your body before an exercise: one standing, one sitting and one lying version. With a relaxed lower abdomen and an erect and agile spine, the energy can travel more easily from the pelvic floor to the brain. A Taoist saying goes: "You will not get any older than your spine is flexible".

Guide exercise 2:

Time: 10 min standing, 5 min sitting, 5 min lying

Purpose: Loosen up and relax your body 💙 Open up the spine 💙 Increase the Qi flow in your body

Preparation: Standing or sitting basic position.

Standing warm-up:

- Shake: feel the connection to mother earth and let a shaking motion come from the ground and bounce up and down from the feet, then from the knees and then from the hips. Shake your shoulders, arms and wrists, each in turn a little extra. Shake your head and then chest, stomach and buttocks. Finally shake the entire body. Stop abruptly and stand still for a while and experience the body.

- Open the hips and chest: guide your pelvis backward by pulling your tailbone in between the legs. Then you slide the pelvis forward and arch the lower back as much as you can. Rock the pelvis back and forth 10 times. Then move in a circular motion 5 turns in each direction, in sequence, first with your tailbone, then the entire pelvis and lastly your chest.

- Spinal cord breathing: bend your arms with your hands in front of your chest. Make soft fists. Breathe in and open your chest and squeeze the shoulder blades by bringing your arms back and shoulders together, arch your lower back forward at the same time, like duck tail. Breathe out, pull the tailbone in between your legs and arch back, the head hangs down slightly, open the shoulder blades, and the arms come together in front of the body. Do this 5 times.

Sitting warm-up:

- Bend the body forward at the hips as far as it goes, until the stomach hits the knees. Roll up vertebra after vertebra, the neck and head comes up last. Do this 5 times.

- Roll down your chin first, then down vertebra after vertebra. Bend the body upwards from the hips. Do 5 times.

- Rock your hip bones from side to side for a minute.

Lying warm-up:

- Lie on your back with your legs bent with the knees towards the ceiling and the feet on the floor. Rock the pelvis rhythmically up and down, by moving the tailbone up and down, and the movement develops through the spine all the way up to the neck. Rock 50 times.

- Lie on your back with stretched legs and arms by the sides. Breathe in and tighten your fists and bend your ankles and push your toes upwards as much as you can. Hold your breath and imagine that you're pushing energy up through your body. Exhale and relax and guide the energy down the spine and down the legs. Do this 3 times.

- Breathe in and fill your chest with air. Hold your breath and push the air down into the abdomen and then back into the chest. Push the air up and down 5 times. Exhale and relax. This provides a massage beneficial for the organs of the abdomen.

- Do the same thing again, but now you breathe in and fill up the abdomen first. Hold your breath and push the air up into the chest and then back down into the abdomen again. Push the air up and down 5 times. Breathe out and relax.

Finishing up, collecting the energy and yin phase

After the exercises that follow, it's fundamental to preserve the energy, the Qi you have generated. You do this by focusing on and laying your hands on Dan Tian. Dan Tian is a neutral place where you can ground your experiences and cultivate your observational ability. The body is given the opportunity to digest the impressions and integrate the exercise. The energy movement that has begun is allowed to be completed. Feel the pulsation of the electromagnetic power. Allow yourself to listen with all your senses and be receptive and sensitive to all the sensations that arise. Going inside awakens the deeper wisdom of your body consciousness. The exercises also end with a so-called yin phase, where you only rest, observe and do nothing. Like meditation in silence, stillness and presence. It's in silence that you can be receptive and listen for answers and hear what you never heard before. The yin phase is important for the balance between activity and receptivity.

Guide exercise 3:

Time: 5 min

Purpose: Deposit energy into your energy account ❤ Ground your experience ❤ Nurture your development of Dan Tian

Gather energy and yin phase:

❧ 1. Put your hands on Dan Tian, just below the navel. Let your attention sink down there and collect the energy. Rest and yin phase. Do nothing, observe, integrate.

If you want to strengthen the gathering effect further, put your left hand on the navel and your right hand on top of the left. Circle your hands clockwise ten turns around the navel, small circles that grow bigger and bigger. Then ten circles counterclockwise, that become smaller and smaller.

The tree, exercise for grounding and inner power

This exercise develops your inner strength and gives you a stable and open body. It helps you to ground yourself in your body and to become more centered and balanced. At the physical level you exercise relaxation, bodily awareness and a good posture. The mind learns concentration and how to be more present. You also nurture your energy body and balance your emotions. When you can hold your whole life experience, you can truly take responsibility of the creational process within you. The more stable the body, the more energy you can cope with. The more relaxed the body is, the more calm and relaxed mind. The more open the body is, the more flow. This you will quickly notice if you practice regularly. When standing in the tree you become conscious of your life force and reunite with your deepest loving nature. The deeper you go inside, the more love will unfold. Your body is waiting for you to move in fully and to be embodied and illuminated by your consciousness.

For devoted Qigong practitioners, there is nothing more exciting than standing still like a tree and observing how the mind behaves facing a feeling or pain. Being able to "sneak" on yourself and feel completely blessed when a tension somewhere in the body will make itself noticed, resolve itself and then release its energy. This process will end up being a fascinating adventure in your own bodily consciousness.

Perineum and the crown

The point in the perineum is called Hui Yin the "Gate of Life and Death" and is situated between the scrotum and the anus. It is a gathering place for yin energies. Through this gate, life energy can easily leak out. You can also let nourishing energy come in from mother earth and nurture you.

The crown is called Bai Hui, the point of "Hundred Convergences" and is situated on top of the head, straight up from the ears. It is linked to the pineal gland and from here you can see the higher perspective and get in touch with father sky.

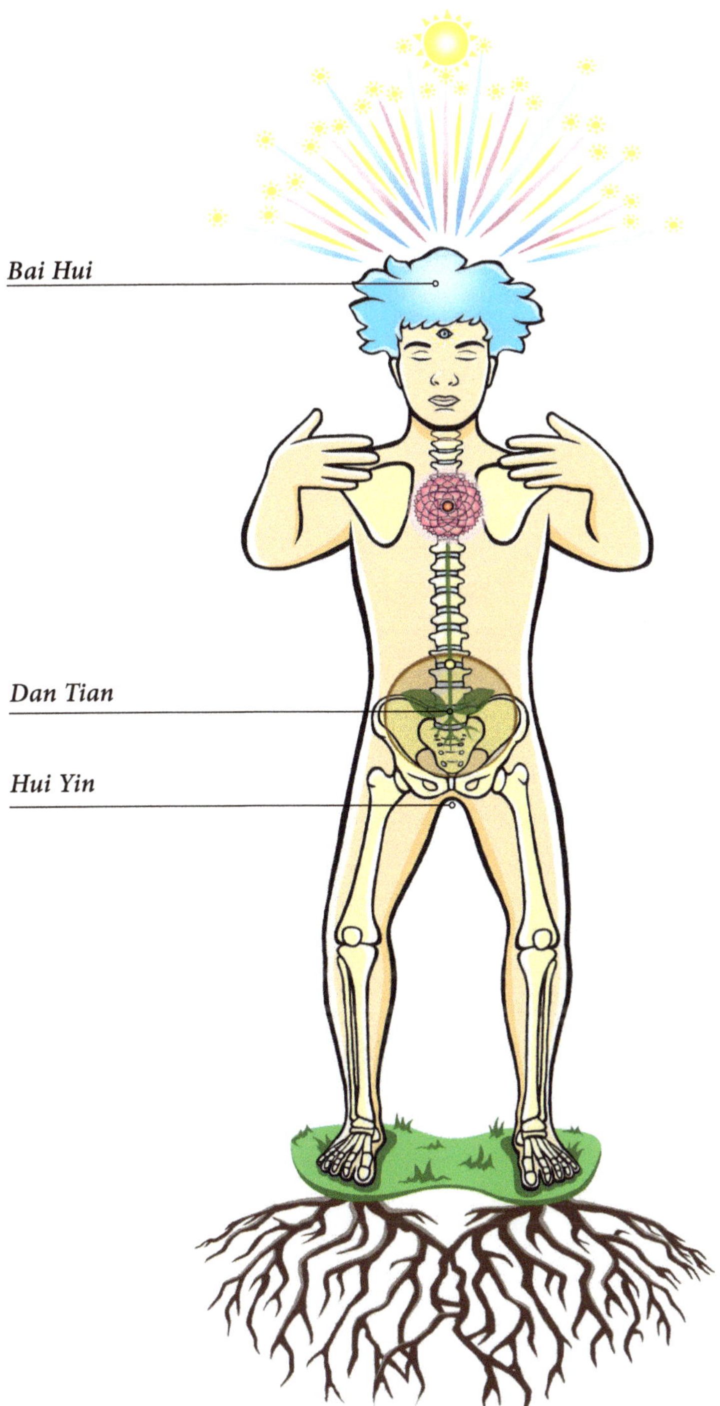

Imagine standing steady like a tree growing towards the light, with your roots deep down in the earth. You receive energy from the sun and receive nourishment from the earth. Feel the connection with both heaven and earth, while being aware of your own body and center, Dan Tian.

Time: 5-15 min

Purpose: To build a stable foundation and ground yourself in your body ❤ Open up to your inner power ❤ Balance yin and yang (earth and sky)

Preparation: Standing basic position and warm-up exercises.

1. Stand in basic position. Bring your hands up in front of you at the height of your neck. Your arms are smoothly rounded as if you were hugging a tree. Your palms are facing you. Slightly spread your fingers. The little fingers point down and towards you and your thumbs up and away from you.

2. Relax the abdomen and buttocks. Imagine grabbing the ground a little extra in with your toes. Let roots grow down into the earth and ground yourself in mother earth. Then feel the connection between the perineum and the earth. Be aware of the crown, the top of the head. Connect with the sky and draw the essence of the sun into your heart.

3. Turn your attention and all your senses inward (see, listen, smell, feel, touch your inside). Relax the mind and breathe calmly and deeply. Guide yourself around within your body. Be aware of unnecessary tension anywhere. Strive to release tensions and open up inside. Correct your posture to the basic position all the time. Observe thoughts and feelings that come and go. Perhaps pain and discomfort transforming into relaxation and pleasure. The aim is to relax more and more while being stable and standing straight.

4. Finish. Put your hands on Dan Tian, move your focus there and collect the energy. Rest and yin phase.

Begin by doing this exercise 5 minutes each time. Increase gradually to 15 minutes. It's recommended to have a mirror to peek at sometimes to correct your posture.

The inner smile

This is one of the classical Taoist meditations. In this exercise you smile in towards yourself and to your internal organs. In this way you activate a pleasant energy, which you can consciously direct to different parts of your body. This meditation develops a sense of acceptance and self-love. It is a deep recognition that there is always an inner smile present, a deep sense of profound inner love. This is a yin opening, where you allow full self-acceptance of all of yourself, and allow yourself to be nourished and rejuvenated.

Andrew Fretwell's take on the inner smile:

Only our essence remains stable at all times. It is a neutral force we all have at our core. The inner smile is the conscious recognition and allowance of this. The inner smile is not something you do, but rather the recognition that at the core of every human being there is a self, that has never been traumatized, and is always free, like an inner sun that is always shining. It's a deep recognition of what is true. Smiling this deep essence into our bodies over time gradually releases all unbalances out of our bodies. We need to address this at the physical dimension of ourselves and it is so much more powerful than meditation alone.

Center of well-being

All 108 muscles of the face are mapped and researchers have come to the conclusion that just by activating the muscles that raise the corners of your mouth and the laughing muscles around the eyes, you affect one of the centers of well-being in the brain, whether you're happy or not. Research on the brain and meditation also confirms that we can change brain activity, and thereby reduce stress and increase well-being. One of the world's leading scientists on mindfulness, David Richardson, has shown that the brain and consciousness are way more plastic than we've previously believed and can change through different techniques and meditation.

The intelligence of the heart

Research has also shown how emotions affect the biochemistry of our bodies. At the HeartMath Institute in California, they have tried to prove the intelligence of the heart. A fact that many indigenous cultures have long been pointing to. They have seen that by shifting our focus from head to heart we can change our attitude and increase the flow of well-being hormones and reduce stress hormones radically. The electromagnetic field of the heart is much stronger than the brain.

See if it works for you by looking at a conflict you have in your life, on your inside or something being played out in your relationships, on the outside. Consider the conflict from the two different perspectives. First from the head, the center of reason and then from the heart, the center of compassion. How does your view and attitude to the conflict change? How do your feelings toward it change? Many people think this sounds way too simple to be true. Try and see if it works for you.

The inner organs

In Chinese medicine, our emotional life and inner organs are connected. The organs in the abdomen have a consciousness and that is where we create and store our feelings. Feelings that you don't want to feel for various reasons do not disappear, but tend to stay inside of you. The energy stagnates and the body becomes tense. Like the food we eat, different experiences need to be digested and processed and we need to learn how to handle all the emotional expressions of being human.

Each yin organ; heart, spleen, lungs, kidneys, liver, has an associated yang organ; small intestine, stomach, large intestine, bladder, gallbladder. If an organ is weak, you may get stuck in negative emotions, and on the contrary, a recurring negative feeling drains the organ. By incorporating a positive feeling you can strengthen the organ. Courage and self-esteem, for example, support the lungs and playfulness is good for the heart. A state of fear or stress drains the kidneys, but can be transformed into care and wisdom. Worry in the spleen has a potential to turn into trust. However, we need all the human emotional expressions, both the negative and positive. Feelings of fear help you to be alert towards danger, anger makes you able to set boundaries etc. According to Tao it is as unhealthy to only feel kindness, as it is to never feel sadness and grief.

In traditional Chinese medicine, the "five element theory" is used to diagnose and describe symptoms and conditions. Water, fire, metal, earth and wood represent different aspects and characteristics and are associated with different organs and senses. Tao believes that all aspects of life can be reflected in the elements. Going out and reflecting yourself in nature is very relaxing and rejuvenating. Hike in the woods, rest on mother earth or on a mountain cliff, listen to a waterfall or look into a fire. Among the most important things we can do is to create an elemental and emotional balance in our lives. In the chart below you can read about how elements, organs, feelings, expressions, colors and senses are connected. You can use the feeling and color of the organ to enhance the effect of your meditation. Stay for a minute or two in each organ. By helping the internal organs to relax, you balance your emotions.

The organs and the "five element theory"

Organ	Kidneys (bladder)	Heart (small intestine)	Lungs (large intestine)	Spleen (stomach, pancreas)	Liver (gall bladder)
Element	water	fire	metal	earth	wood
Color	blue	red	white	yellow	green
Negative emotion	fear, stress	malice, arrogance, impatience	sadness, depression, grief	mental worry, stress	anger, aggression, frustration
Positive emotion	caution, awareness, wisdom, stillness	love, playfulness, joy, enthusiasm	strength, courage, integrity, independence	stability, centering, compassion	kindness, generosity
Expression	life-force and the desire to live	to be able to give and receive	ability to let go and devote yourself	to have trust and a relaxed mind	will power, making decisions, creativity, expansion
Physical	regulate bodily fluids and blood pressure, purify the blood	pumps the blood	inhaling oxygene and exhaling carbomonoxid	filters the blood, supports immune system	assimilating nutrition and detoxing the blood
Position	by the lower back, close to the spine	in the chest, slightly to the left	in the chest	below the ribs to the left	partly below the ribs to the right
Sense	ears, hearing	tongue, speech	nose, smell	lips, taste	eyes, vision

Time: 10 min

Purpose: Transform negative energy into vitality ❤ Balance your organs and emotions ❤ Create an accepting inner atmosphere

Preparation: Sitting basic position.

1. Create a smile on your lips. Think of someone you like, a child, an animal, a place, something that really makes you smile. Then let go of the image and direct the smile inwards.

2. Direct your attention and the smile to your genitals. Sink down and guide your breath there. Really feel the connection and awaken of the energy.

3. Then move your attention and smile to your kidneys. Breathe down into the kidneys. How are your kidneys doing? Feel and listen to them. Make them relax. Feel stillness and gentleness. Let the kidneys bathe in blue light.

4. Now move your attention to the liver and direct your smile there. Guide your breathing there, watch and listen. Feel a sense of kindness and generosity. Allow the liver to be filled with green light.

5. Then move the attention and the smile to your heart. Guide your breathing there, feel, look down, and listen to your heart. Maybe your heart is smiling back at you. Feel a sense of joy, love and playfulness and let the heart be filled with a red light.

6. Then move your attention to the spleen. Smile down to your spleen and guide your breathing there. Let the mind relax. Feel a sense of trust and stability and fill the spleen with a yellow light.

7. Then move the attention to the lungs. Smile at them and guide your breath and your awareness there. Feel self-esteem, courage and strength. Breathe in a white light into the lungs.

8. In the end, go back to the kidneys and then guide all the energy you have created to Dan Tian.

9. Finish. Put your hands on Dan Tian, move your focus there and collect the energy. Rest and yin phase.

The order follows the positive cycle of the five element theory of traditional Chinese medicine, where the elements support and nurture each other. The fire gives nutrition (ashes) to the earth, the earth produces metal, metal gives nutrients (minerals) to the water, the water nurtures the tree, and wood gives fuel to the fire. Examples of the negative cycle are metal that cuts down the tree or water that puts out the fire. Usually, only the nurturing cycle is used for internal exercises.

The inner organs

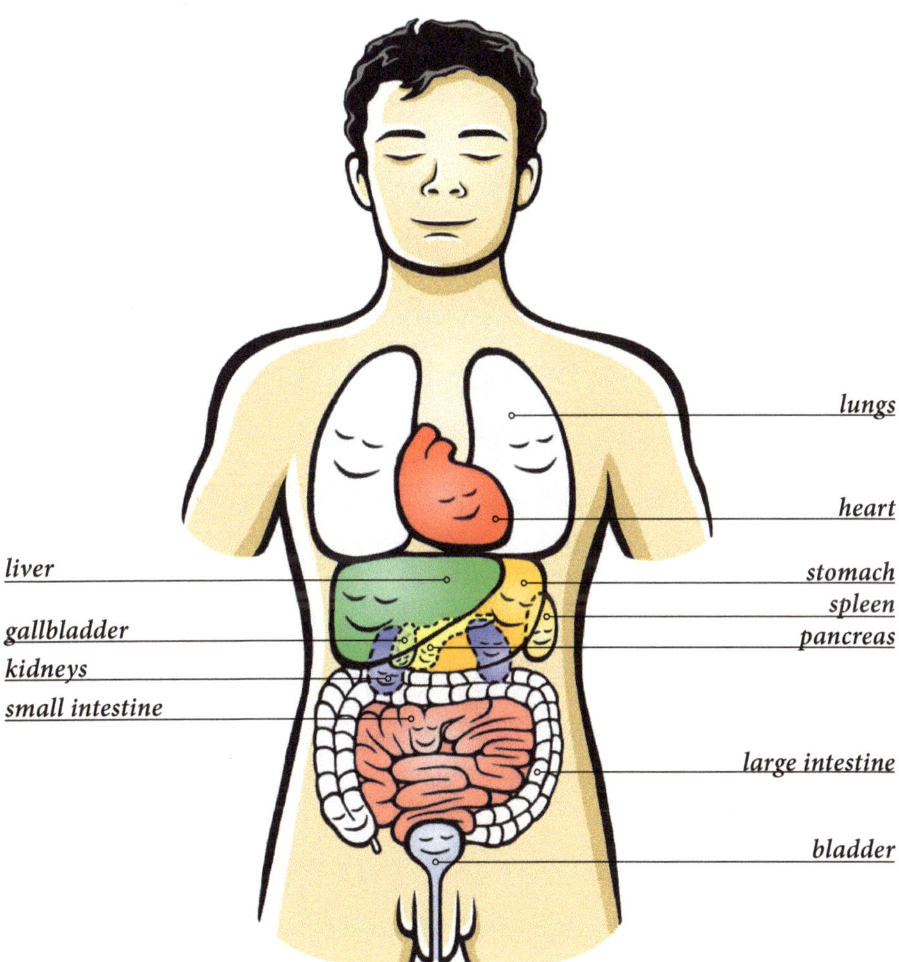

In Chinese medicine emotions and organs are connected. The organs have a consciousness and are where feelings are created and stored. By helping the organs relax you're making them happy and you're also supporting your emotional balance.

The short inner smile

Feel free to do this shorter version before exercises in connection with the basic positions. It will put you in a state of deeper presence and a positive atmosphere. It's a simple, effective and soothing exercise that you can, in principle, perform anywhere and at any time.

Guide Exercise 6:

Time: 5 min

Purpose: Turn your focus inward ❤ Create a state of presence ❤ Develop an attentive and peaceful attitude

Preparation: Sitting or standing basic position.

1. Imagine a person that you really like (or child, animal, nature) who laughs and has a warm and welcoming smile to you.

2. Receive the smile and absorb it through your 3rd eye.

3. Let the smile penetrate your brain.

4. Then direct the smile down to your heart. Guide your breath there and really feel the connection and awaken the energy. Fall into the void of your heart. Feel, look into and listen to your heart.

5. Then drop down your awareness into your center. Smile down at Dan Tian and the lower abdomen. Include your genitals. Feel and awaken subtle exited energy and let your life force expand.

6. Then guide the energy and the smile up the spine and through the nervous system, throughout your body. Let the smile penetrate every cell and make them energized and happy.

7. Finish. Put your hands on Dan Tian and rest for a short while.

Now you are in a good state to move on with other exercises or take on everyday life.

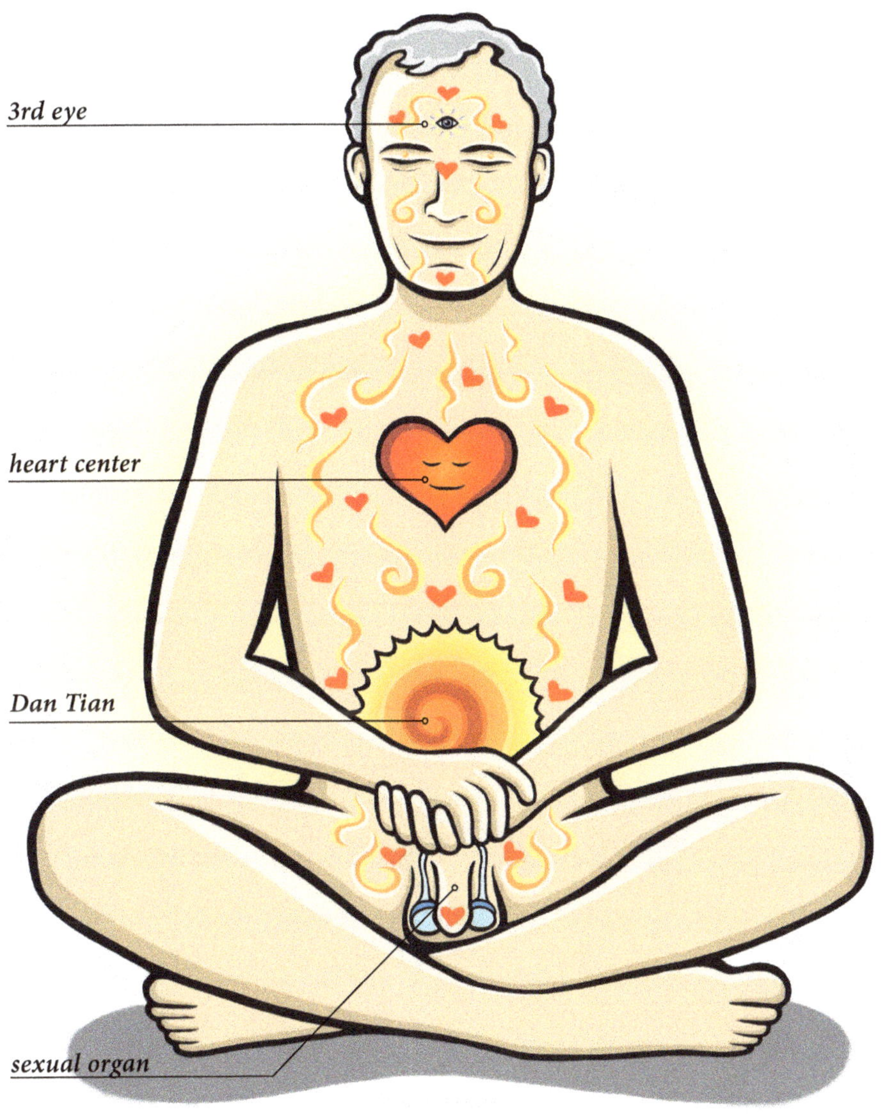

The inner smile creates a positive and loving inner atmosphere.

EXERCISE 7:

The small circulation

The small circulation (SC) is an exercise where you circulate, transform and distribute energy. Being able to know and guide Qi through different centers and meridians in the body is the very foundation of Taoist energy work. In SC, the energy is circulated along the two central meridians, Du Mai (yang) that goes up the spine and Ren Mai (yin) that goes down the front. The channels help regulate the flow of yin and yang energy in the other 12 organ-related meridians. The Qi is then spread throughout the body. One purpose of Qigong is specifically to create a fresh energy flow in these "rivers" of Qi. SC also links important energy points and energy centers. When Qi is allowed to flow freely in the SC the entire body is nurtured and harmonized. The life energy is cleared and refined. You get a strong and resilient body and a clear and flexible mind. Work with this circulation is not only done within Tao, but also in several other traditions.

Du Mai and Ren Mai

Du Mai starts in the perineum (between the scrotum and anus) and rises along the spine, to the base of the skull and the crown, then down through the point between the eyebrows and ends in your palate. Ren Mai takes over the circulation through the tongue and goes down the front and ends in the perineum. You place the tip of your tongue up on the palate to tie the two meridians together and ground the energy in the body. The channels pass about a centimeter into the body. The points are inputs to energy centers in the body.

Taoist mystic says: *In the beginning there was only the void, WuJi, which holds the potential of all things. In the creation, when egg (yin) and sperm (yang) met and attached to the uterus wall, the attachment became Chi Hai (navel) and the opposite became Ming Men (lower back). From Chi Hai, Ren Mai (water) was created and from Ming Men, Du Mai (fire) was created and in the middle emerged the third channel Chong Mai. From this, the 10,000 things emerged.*

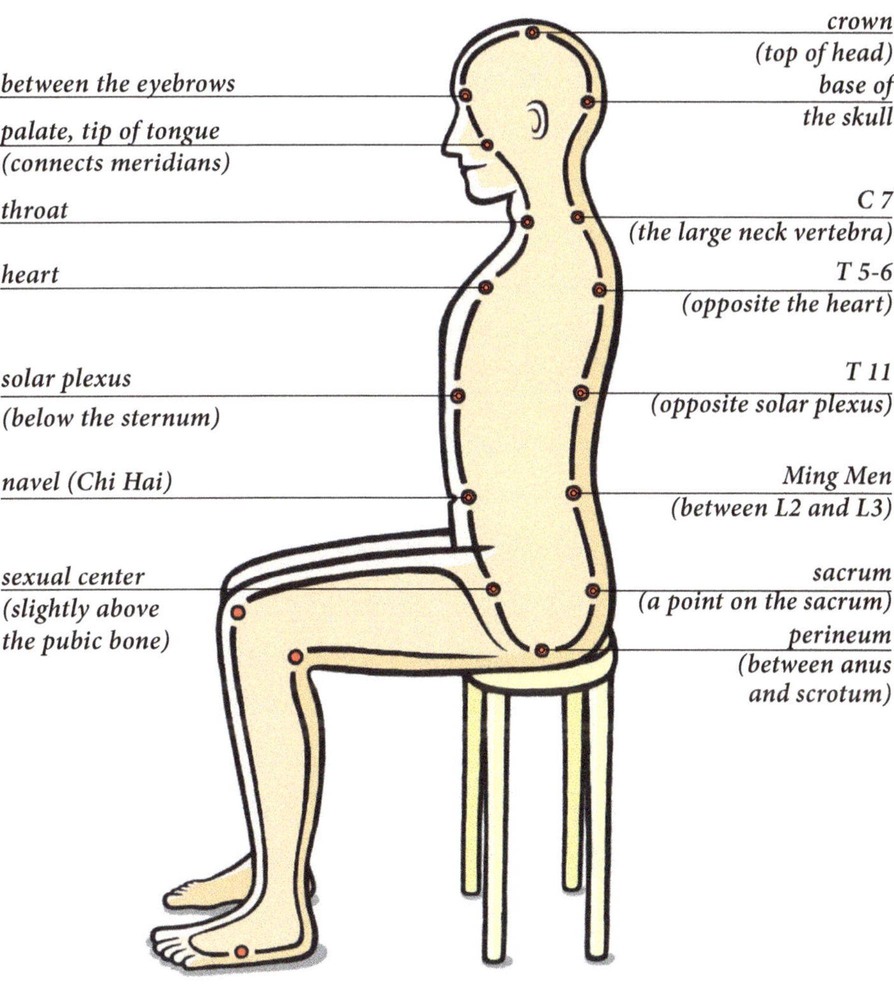

To open this circulation fully is a lifetime project with full enlightenment as a goal. So have perseverance and enjoy the ride along the way.

Explore the points

You connect with and open the points by directing your attention and a smile towards each point. Breathe in and out into the point. Also strengthen the connection with the help of a clear focus and using your inner eyes and ears. Be present and let your awareness touch every point. Feel how the points open up and relax. Experience, explore and perceive each and every point. Does it feel relaxed or blocked? What is it like to focus on each point? Or looking out at the world or perceiving the world from there? Does it feel comfortable or unpleasant? Is there a lot of energy or a small amount of energy? Are there any distinctions between the different points?

Stay longer at the points in the back, preferably a few minutes on each. On the front, the energy flows like a waterfall and touches the points on the way down. The more the points open, the easier it becomes to circulate the energy in SC. Eventually you'll be able to do a whole round in one breath.

At first, it may be difficult to concentrate on and feel the points. But it usually gets better over time. One effect, and many agree with me, is that a nice relaxed feeling is created in the body as energy begins to flow and the mind becomes more peaceful, open and relaxed.

Through your mind you can lead Qi to any part of the body. You first develop the sensitivity to feel each part of the body internally. Important is as well to really feel the Qi. The deeper the mind reaches in the meditations the more profound and effective this practise will be. You can trust that your presence will make a difference.

Guide exercise 7:

Time: 15 min

Purpose: Circulate Qi and provide the body with life energy ❤ Open, activate and connect different energy centers in the body ❤ Unravel physical and mental blockages

Preparation: Sitting basic position, sitting warm-up and a short inner smile.

1. Focus and breathe into Dan Tian. Go deep inside behind and below the navel. Sink down.

2. Breathe in and imagine pulling the energy from Dan Tian down to the next point, the sexual center above the pubic bone. Breathe out at this point.

3. Breathe in and imagine pulling the energy down from the sexual center to the next point, perineum, between the anus and the scrotum. Breathe out and stay in the perineum. Rest, explore and breathe in and out of the point in the perineum.

4. Then inhale into the perineum and guide the energy up to the next point, at the center of the sacrum. Breathe out and stay at this point. Rest, explore and breathe in and out through the sacrum.

5. Continue in the same way to move the energy up to the entire spine and go through each point. Ming Men, opposite the navel, T11, opposite solar plexus, T5, between the shoulder blades, C7, the neck, base of the skull and the crown, top off the head. Rest in the crown for a moment.

6. Then put the tip of the tongue on the palate and guide the energy faster down the front, between the eyebrows, through the tongue down the throat, the heart point, solar plexus, the navel, the sexual center and finally the perineum. Rest in the perineum for a while.

7. Now breathe in and drag the energy through all the points, up the spine, hold your breath and focus a few seconds on the crown. Then exhale, and let the energy flow down through the points on the front side. Keep the tip of your tongue against your palate all the time.

8. Circle the energy 10 turns. One round per breath.

9. Finish. Put your hands on Dan Tian, keep your focus there and collect the energy. Rest and yin phase.

Testicle massage

The testicles are central to a man's production of sex hormones, especially testosterone. By massaging your testicles you help the testicles to release tension and increase blood circulation. You also support the connection with your sexual essence. The testicles are directly connected to both your brain and genitals via the endocrine system and contain a multitude of small glands. Massage your testicles often and with delight to keep them healthy. Stretching the whole genital package releases tension in the root of the penis and reinforces the circulation of Qi. Keep testicle massage and stretching apart from masturbation.

Testicular massage

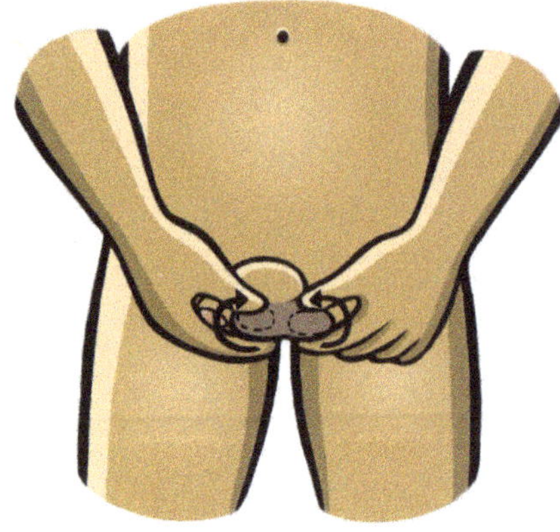

Massage by circulating outwards and then inwards

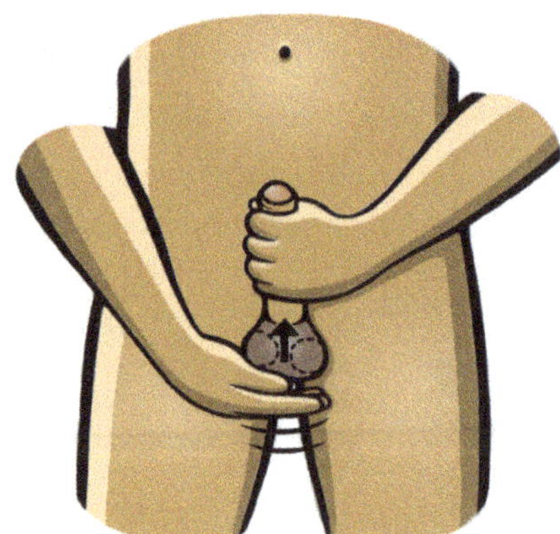

Bump your scrotum up and down

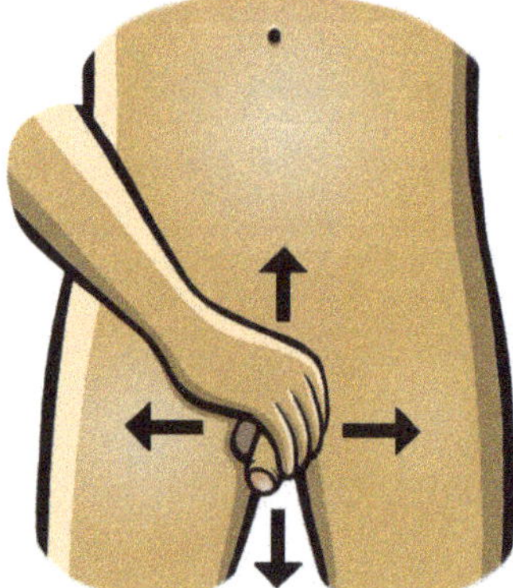

Hold the root of the penis and stretch in the different directions

Connect with your testicles from within, how are they feeling? Give them your attention, acceptance and gratefulness for the life force and joy they give you. Regular massages can prevent imbalances and keep them relaxed and vital.

116

Guide exercise 8:

Time: 5-10 min

Purpose: Strengthen sexual power ♥ Increase circulation ♥ Give appreciation

Preparation: Sitting basic position.

1. Sit on the edge of your chair (with loose pants, or without pants at all).

2. Rub your hands warm.

3. Hold both testicles with your hands and feel the warmth from your hand.

4. Direct your breath and attention to your testicles, smile at them and go there with your awareness. Experience them from the inside. Give them appreciation and feel gratitude.

5. Hold each testicle between your thumbs and fingers on each hand. They feel a lot like little apricots. Then gently massage 10 turns outwards and then 10 turns inwards. Circle and press in different places.

6. Hold your penis with one hand and bump your scrotum up and down with the fingers of the other hand for about one minute.

7. Take a steady grip of the penis and the scrotum, by the root of the penis. Use your thumb and forefinger on one hand.

8. Pull the penis forward and simultaneously tighten the pelvic floor muscles for a few seconds. Repeat left, right, up and down.

9. Sit still and feel the energy rise up in the body. The yin phase is essential for receiving, digesting and integrating the energy movement created by the exercise.

The penis root attaches to the bulbospongiosus and ischiocavernosus muscles about 2 inches into the body (see picture on p. 132). The muscles can be stretched and exercised to promote a stronger erection, create greater control over ejaculation and a more intense orgasm. The practice is also said to be able to extend the limb slightly.

A similar exercise is sometimes called the "deer exercise". Long ago, Taoists discovered that some animals lived for a long time. One of these was the deer who also had a strong sexual drive. They carefully studied the behaviors which gave the deer its characteristics. From there came these exercises into being, where testicle massage was combined with activating the pelvic floor and guiding the energy into the body.

Charge your life energy

This exercise will revitalize your kidneys, testicles and Dan Tian. The kidneys are placed deep inside the body, quite high up in your lower back. It is about where the lumbar spine meets the thoracic spine, adjacent to and in front of the spine. The kidneys are seen as the batteries of the body and are very important to support your life force energy, vitality and libido. Your original, raw power (Jing) is stored in the kidneys. In this exercise you will charge your life energy by combining stimulation of your kidneys, testicles and navel. It will increase your energy and well-being.

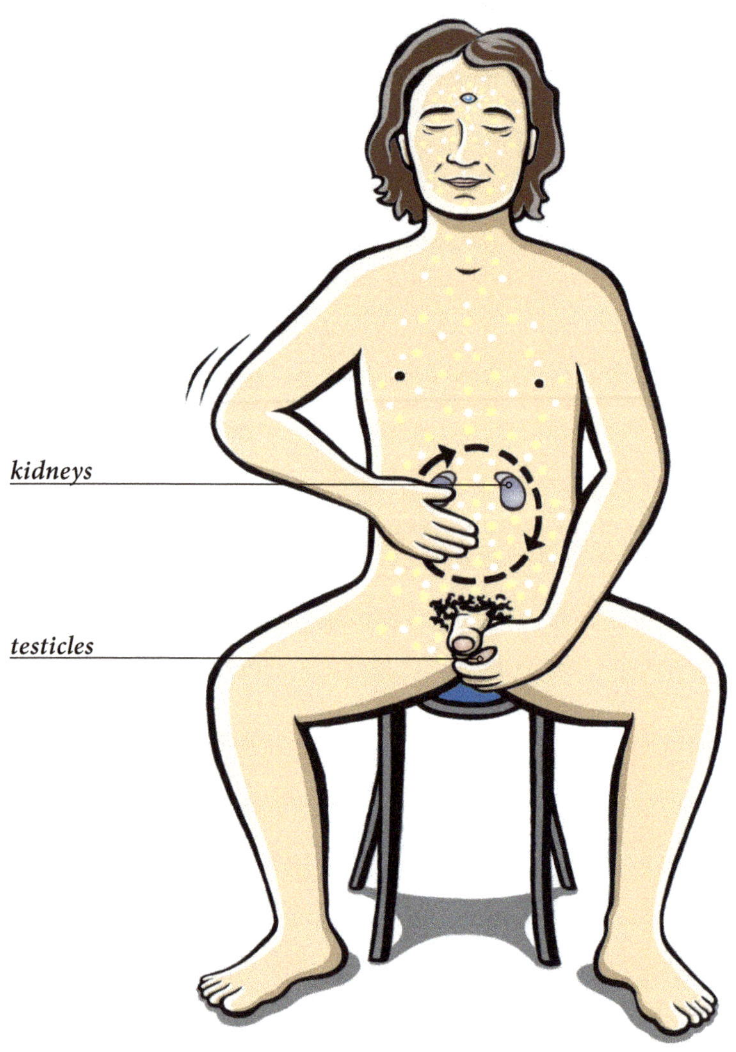

Time: 10 min

Purpose: Activate Dan Tian ❤ Connect the different parts ❤ Awaken life energy

Preparation: Sitting basic position and a short inner smile.

1. Rub your hands warm.

2. Put your tongue up against the palate.

3. Hold the testicles between thumbs and fingers on each hand.

4. Gently massage the testicles 10 turns outwards and 10 turns inwards.

5. Pause, turn your focus towards the sexual center.

6. Move your hands to your kidneys.

7. Massage the kidneys. Rub with your fingers or the back of your hand up and down.

8. Pause, focus on Ming Men.

9. Hold the testicles with your left hand. Feel the heat from your hand. Place your right hand slightly above the pubic bone. Feel the heat from your hand. Massage clockwise 10 big circles around the navel.

10. Pause, focus deep inside your Dan Tian.

11. The hands change place, the right hand holds the testicles and the left hand is placed just above the pubic bone. Massage counterclockwise 10 big circles around the navel.

12. Pause, focus and breathe deep into the middle of Dan Tian, include awareness of the pelvic floor. Sit and rest for a while, with your hands placed in each other.

13. Continue with testicle breathing and/or circulate energy in the SC.

14. Or just finish and collect the energy, put your hands on Dan Tian and rest, yin phase.

Testicle breathing

Every day, millions of sperm and sex hormones are produced in your testicles. Each sperm contains the opportunity to create new life. According to Taoism, the sperms hold the essence of your vitality, your yang nature, your DNA and your Jing energy. To awaken and use this slumbering power, they created testicle breathing. The exercise stimulates the production of hormones and makes use of the essential energy of the sperms and transforms it into life force energy.

The activated potency of the sperms and the sexual energy in a subtly excited state is guided in SC. The Jing energy needs to be circulated and refined for your body to be able to absorb it. Sexual energy is a raw material that needs to be transformed. As the energy is transported through the spine, it becomes refined and can thus be used by the brain and is easier taken care of by the body. This exercise is sometimes called "the fountain of youth" and has several beneficial effects.

The essence of the sperm and aroused energy

So, in testicle breathing, you make use of the essence of the sperm and subtle orgasmic energy. You can proceed with this exercise and practice by yourself with more excited and hot orgasmic energy. It's then important that the channels are open for the energy to move in SC without excessive blockages. Once you've been training yourself, you can also move forward with a partner. But it is by yourself that you exercise best, not in the heat of the moment. Take your time to practice and learn to know and feel your own sexual essence. You can use aroused energy to charge your body with health and well-being. Gradually you learn to direct energy with only your intention, but until then, use the technique to train and guide the energy. It will pay off.

Cultivation with partner

If you have a partner, you can circulate the energy into two circles that intersect. You receive your partner's energy through the tongue, guide it down the front of your body and transfer it to the partner again through your genitals. It then goes up your partner's spine and back to you. At the same time, your partner receives your energy through her tongue, and down her front channel, into your genitals and then the energy goes up through your spine again. The energy moves in an eight between both of you (see picture on p. 61).

This is how Andrew Fretwell, teacher of Taoist sexual practice, describes the value of testicle breathing and testicle massage:

There are so many good things with the Tao training. When you do a testicle massage you increase your testosterone levels, which in turns makes your erection harder and has many benefits for your health. But if you really want to be a better lover, I believe in practicing both testicle massage and testicle breathing. Both of these exercises strengthen your yin, while your yang automatically grows. You cultivate your receptivity and creativity while awakening and guiding your amazing creational power from your testicles out through the body and up to the brain. It's an incredible source of nutrition. The second thing that happens when you begin dedicating yourself to testicle breathing is that you become irresistible to women. Most men are looking for deep relaxation, deepest yin. Therefore, they become frenetic and stressed when they find that women have what they are looking for. When you start doing testicle breathing and performing testicle massage, you begin to strengthen the yin in yourself. This makes you less dependent on women, and women find this attractive. By cultivating yin, you become more appealing to women. The important thing is that you do the exercise, that you stay present and feel what is happening within you. The testicle breathing connects yourself with your life purpose and helps you to find your meaning by increasing your contact with your yin nature. You begin to realize yourself and become more self-sufficient, even sexually. Being able to be enough in yourself is the ultimate spirituality.

The fountain of youth

Beneficial sex hormones with associated feelings are produced in your body every day. Even when you get slightly aroused or excited, the intensity increases. Tao calls the hormones the "fountain of youth", a power and happiness you can have access to every day. Once you understand this and are free to feel your desire and can circulate your sexual energy, you can basically make use of it anywhere and any time.

Note!

If you are worried and stressed, make sure that you have the ability to ground yourself before doing testicle breathing.

In testicle breathing, you skip the back heart point and Ming Men. The heart because it's easy to get too much heat there and Ming Men since it is in itself a transformation point for sexual energy. Once you feel that the energy is refined you can incorporate all the points and circulate it in SC.

Time: 15 min

Purpose: Refine, transform and guide the sexual energy, Jing ❤ Strengthen your receptivity and awaken your creational force ❤ Nurture hormone and nervous systems and brain

Preparation: Sitting basic position, sitting warm-up, testicle massage.

1. Direct your attention towards the genitals, especially the testicles.

2. Breathe in and squeeze the pelvic floor muscles softly and feel the testicles as you squeeze. Breathe out through the testicles and relax. Keep breathing in this way until the area is filled with energy. Note which squeezing that activates the most energy, subtle, soft, light, sucking, sensual etc. (see various pelvic floor exercises on p. 134).

3. Now you should guide the energy from the testicles to different points in the back. You do this by simultaneously squeezing, inhaling and pulling the energy from the testicles to the next point. Then breathe out at the point, relax and fill it with the energy. Go straight back to the testicles and breathe in, squeeze and move the energy upwards. Do about 3 pulls at each point, or continue until the point feels filled with energy.

4. The first point you guide the energy to is the perineum. Then continue on to the sacrum, T11, C7, the base of the skull and the crown. You draw the energy all the way from the testicles and up the spine to the respective point, on one breath and one squeeze. Breathe out into the point.

5. After filling the crown you keep your attention there and circulate the energy just above the crown three times clockwise, then three times counterclockwise. Also let the eyes "look around" the crown inside your inner world. You breathe in and softly hold your breath at the same time.

6. Then let the energy flow down, while breathing out, like a waterfall on the front of your body along the frontal meridian, point by point, but now faster. The tongue is up against your palate.

7. Then circulate the energy in SC. First, you can go around a turn, point by point and now also include Ming Men and the back heart point, T5. Then you can pull the energy around on one and the same breath. Breathing in, bring the energy up the spine, and breathing out, bring the energy down the front line. Let the energy circle 10 turns.

122

8. Finish. Put your hands on Dan Tian, move your focus there and collect the energy. Rest and yin phase.

9. Sit or lie down and just rest, let the body integrate the energy, 5-10 minutes.

Testicle breathing

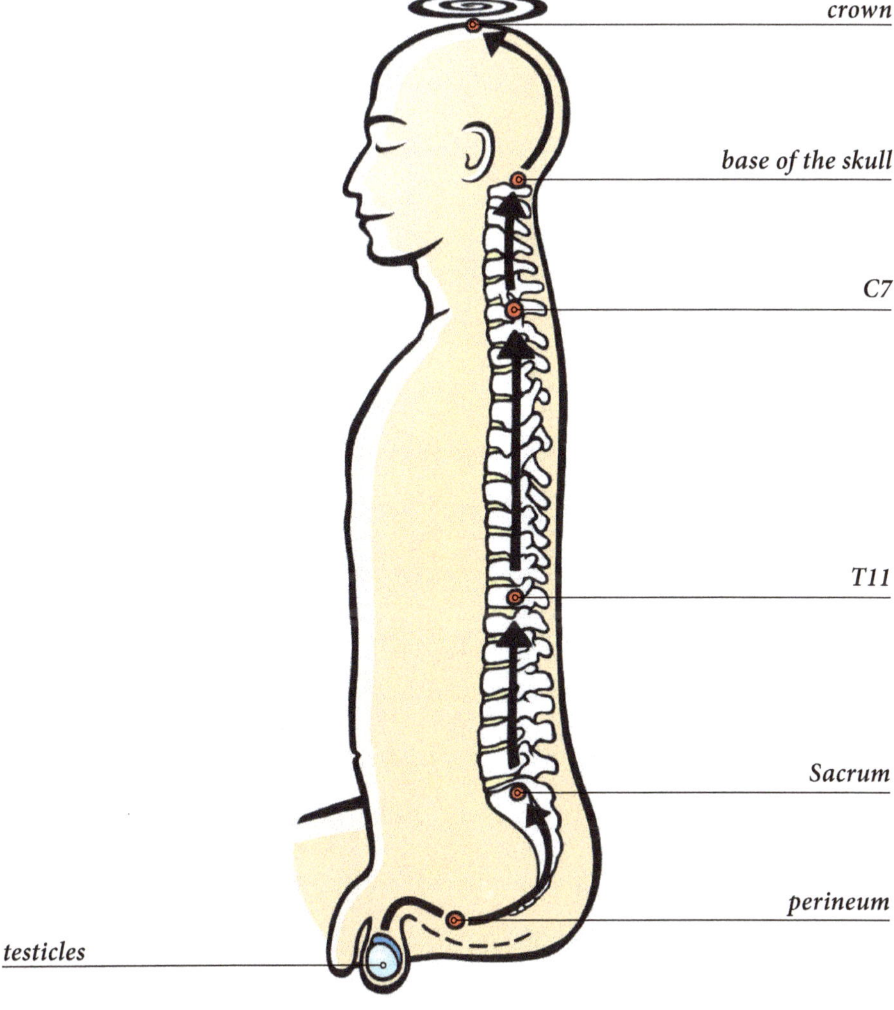

In testicle breathing you practice your ability to deepen your connection to your sexual essence and guide energy up your spine. You activate both your receptivity (yin) and your creativity (yang).

EXERCISE 11:

Hormone shower

The word hormone means to "awaken to life" or movement. The endocrine glands produce these governing chemical substances, which transmit signals with the blood to different parts of the body. Hormones affect multiple functions, including blood pressure, metabolism, genital functions, blood sugar levels and energy supply. Their function is crucial to our development and well-being.

Entries to other worlds

Our seven big glands (see picture on p. 127) are important centers in the body with different tasks. They regulate the energy supply between different body parts as well as balancing each other internally. If one of the glands weakens or is overstimulated, it will affect the others. Each gland can also be assigned different qualities independent of their hormone production and is seen as a gateway to another reality. By activating the glands, their hidden powers can be awakened. They will become a guide to deep transformational experiences. You awaken them by strengthening your contact with them and by feeling them from the inside.

The glands correspond with the chakras, just like in yoga, as well as with the points you opened in the small circulation. Balancing and raising the energy level in the glands is an important part of the Taoist way of developing, healing and strengthening the physical body. Moreover the immune system gets stimulated and reinforces the cells, the building blocks of our body. Tao connects the hormones with our Jing energy. When the energy is transformed you will shine, and an energy of vitality is produced that is very refreshing. Described below are the various characteristics of the glands and briefly their functions and hormone production. Then an exercise follows to increase the equilibrium in the endocrine system.

The pineal gland: The place of spirit
Attributes: Epiphysis, or "soul dwelling" as it is sometimes called, helps you to get in touch with the spiritual, to surrender to the great consciousness. It's like an antenna, it can send and receive messages. Guiding you to the light. Control the other glands.
Physical function: Control cycles, day rhythm and perception of light through eyes and skin.
Hormones: Oxytocin, serotonin, melatonin, DMT, pinoline.
Located: Large as half a pea and situated on the roof of the middle brain, located at the rear edge of the third ventricle and attached to the thalamus.

The pituitary gland: The place of intelligence

Attributes: Helps you develop your psyche and your autonomy. The way to wisdom and the memory of who you are. Visions, compassion, devotion.

Physical function: Regulates growth, reproduction, water and mineral balance. Managing director of the other glands.

Hormone: Oxytocin, prolactin, controls secretion of sex hormones.

Located: Behind the eyebrows, on a branch of the hypothalamus. About as large as a pea.

The thyroid gland: The place of growth

Attributes: Supports you to continue searching, growing and developing. The gateway to your ability to be open minded and the experience of meaningfulness.

Physical function: Affects metabolism in all cells of the body and regulates body temperature. The thyroid glands regulate calcium metabolism in your bones.

Hormone: Thyroxine (T4, T3).

Located: In front of and on both sides of the trachea, and on the back are four small parathyroid glands.

The thymus gland: The place of heart

Attributes: Sometimes called the rejuvenation gland. Guides you to the highest form of love. Also teaches us about creativity, playfulness, talent, beauty and harmony.

Physical function: The thymus gland is very active during the growth phase of puberty. It is also important for the immune system.

Hormone: Thymosin, T-cells (white blood cells that is part of body's immune system).

Located: Behind the breastbone just above the heart and is about 2x1,5x0,2 inches.

The pancreas: The place of transformation

Attributes: Supports transformation and integration of emotions. Guides you from control and power to trust and compassion.

Physical function: Digestion, regulates sugar metabolism.

Hormone: Insulin and glucagon.

Located: Partially behind the stomach and on the left, just below the ribs. It is elongated and about 5-6 inches long.

The adrenal glands: The place of water and fire

Attributes: Provides nutrition and energy to your kidneys, genitals, bone marrow and spine. Reinforces strength and awareness to both mental development and physical training.

Physical function: Associated with the nervous system, brain, bone marrow. The adrenal glands also produce substances that are vital to the body's metabolism of minerals, trace elements, carbohydrates, fat and protein.

Hormone: Produces the stress hormones cortisol and adrenaline and the feel good hormone DHEA, and aldosterone, progesterone, estrogen, testosterone.

Located: The kidneys are approximately the size of your ears and the adrenals are located on top of them like small triangular hats. Situated close to the spine approximately between L2 and T11.

The testicles: The place of essence

Attributes: Provides vigor for your genitals and sexuality.

Physical function: Produces sperm and male sex hormones. Important for genital development, muscles, skeletons, libido.

Hormone: DHEA, testosterone.

Located: Size varies, but about the size of an apricot. Situated in the scrotum.

The thrusting channel

During the exercise "hormone shower" you will guide the energy through the thrusting channel, Chong Mai, which goes like a tube through the body. It goes from the perineum, up through the prostate, and all the way up to the brain. Along the way, the channel affects the glands and thus the chakras -the energy centers in the body - through which we experience, engage with, and perceive the world. These need to be open, but also in contact with each other for a full life experience. A chakra activity that is too low or too high results in an inharmonic and unbalanced individual. Each energy center affects one or more glands and, in addition, different organs as well as the mind's mood.

The gateway of origin

The mouth of the prostate opens into the urethra. The opening is an important point called Guan Yuan, which means the "gate of origin". It's like a gateway that you can go through, in or out. It normally opens outwards during ejaculation and urination. During the female orgasm, the Guan Yuan point (cervix) opens inward, therefore, in contrast to the man, the women do not lose as much energy during the orgasm. By changing the direction of male's sexual flow, from going outward, to going inward, males can make use of their original life energy. You open this gateway in the hormone shower exercise by guiding energy through the thrusting channel. View it as exploring your and your life's origin. Through this exercise you also stimulate and refill your life force energy.

The different glands work together in a very elegant and ingenious way. The hormone system is central to many functions of the body. Therefore you always go through all the glands when doing this exercise. It is very important to rest afterwards and allow the

The seven large endocrine glands and hypothalamus and thalamus

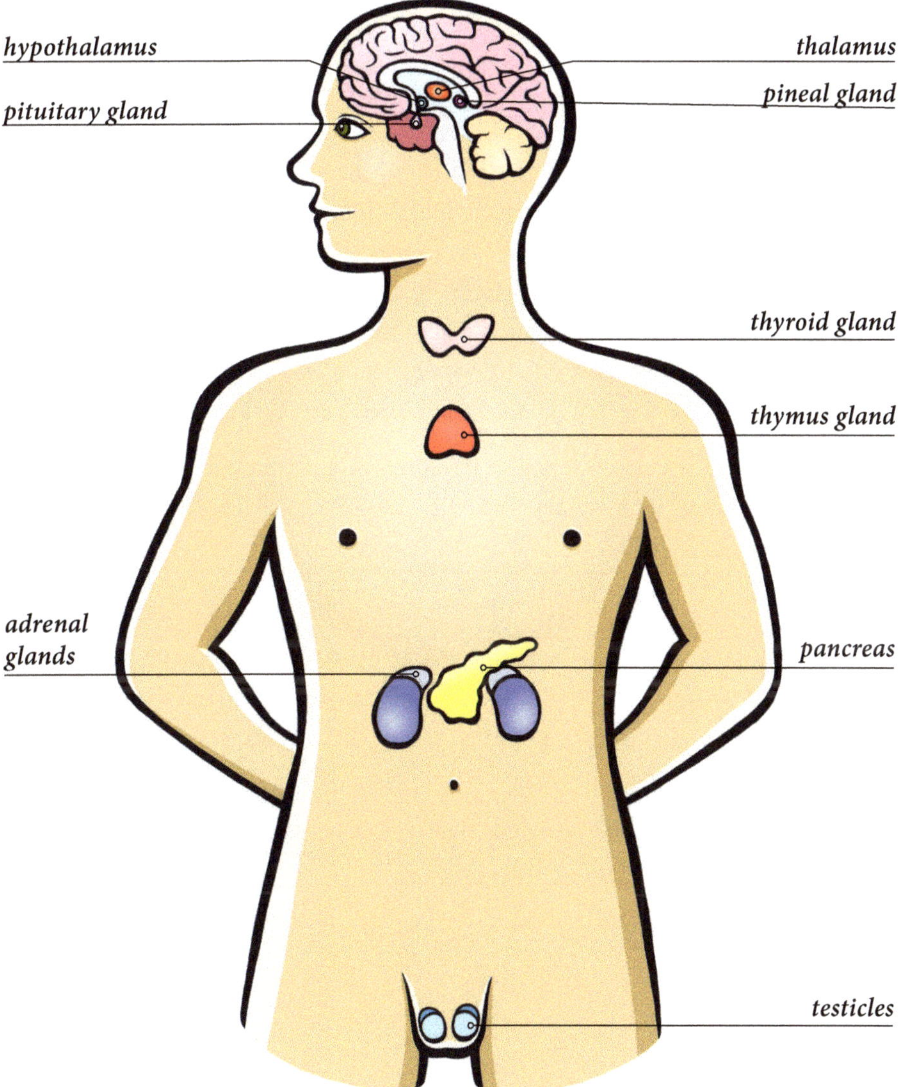

The endocrine glands may be assigned different qualities and are perceived as the gateways to other worlds. The awakening of the glands will increase your well-being and deepen your life experience.

body to integrate the impact. This is an exercise with a very strong and balancing influence. I can't emphasize enough the importance of the yin phase and to enjoy the potential healing and peace afterwards.

Guide exercise 11:

Time: 20 min
Purpose: Connect with and explore the glands 💜 Balance the hormone system 💜 Bind the energy centers together

Preparation: Sitting basic position, warm-up exercises and/or short inner smile.

1. Direct your attention to your testicles and stay there. Give them an inner smile to establish a connection. Let your smile, breath, presence and consciousness sink down to and touch your testicles. Look inside with your inner eyes, listen with your inner ears, and explore what it's like to be present there. Does it feel relaxed or blocked? Can you loosen up and soften? Maybe you will perceive images and messages, or perhaps not. It doesn't matter what. Your presence will still affect and stimulate the area. Maybe as an inner subtle massage of your testicles.

2. Continue to do the same thing with the adrenal glands, the pancreas, the thymus, the thyroid gland, the pituitary gland and the pineal gland. Stay for at least a few minutes on each gland.

3. As you have gone through all glands, you place your focus down at the perineum.

4. Then breathe in and guide the energy up into the middle of the body, into Chong Mai, the thrusting channel, which touches all the glands and chakras on the way up.

5. Breathe out through the top of your head and let the energy spray like a fountain and shower yourself with this sparkling hormone energy. Go down to the perineum again and breathe likes this 3-6 times.

6. Finally lay down and rest fully for at least 10 minutes.

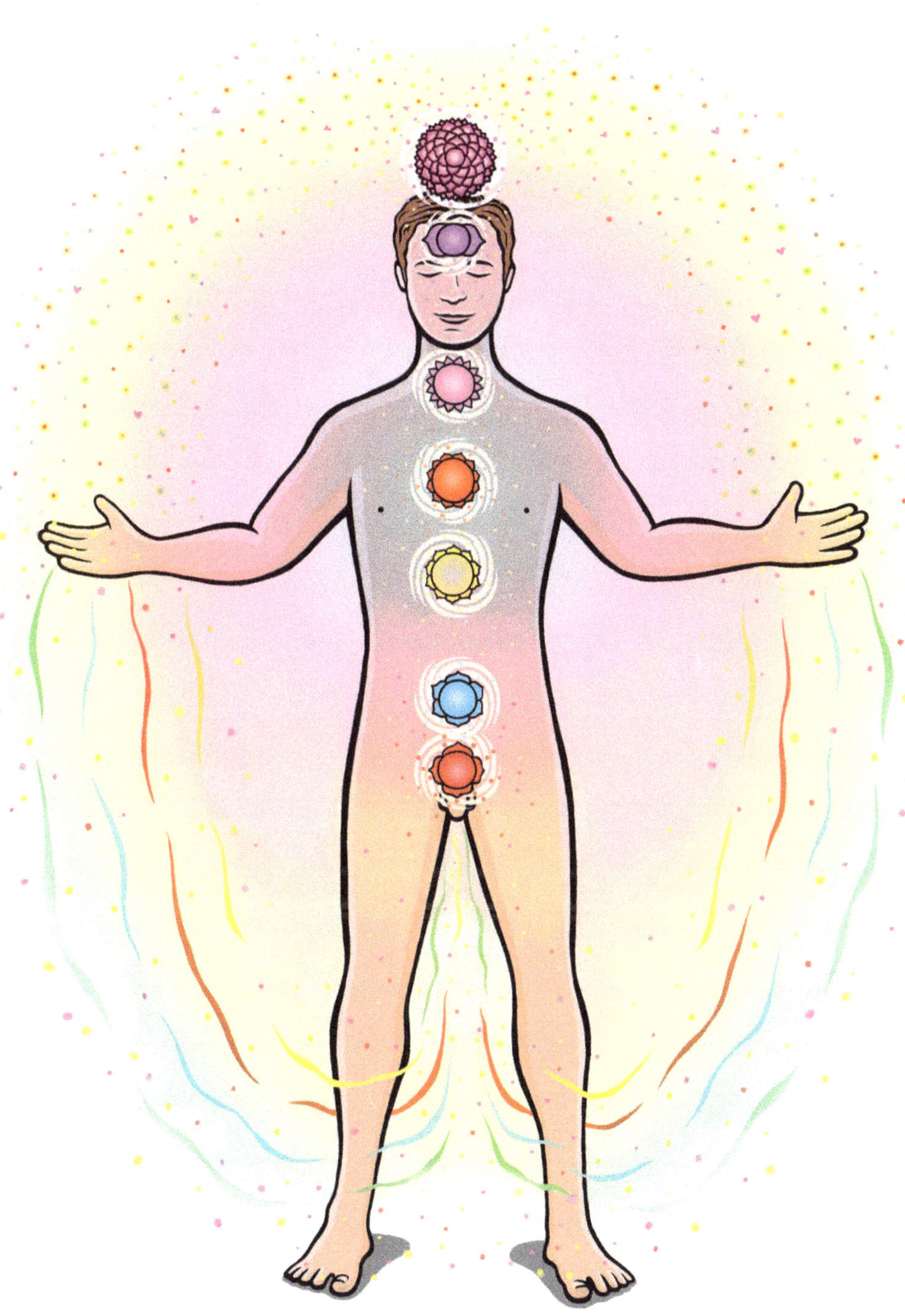

In the exercise "hormone shower" you guide the energy up through Chong Mai, which goes up the middle of your body and touches the glands and chakras.

Squeezing exercises

Pelvic floor muscles

The pelvic floor is made up of different, overlapping layers of muscles and fascia. They can be resembled to several hammocks suspended in different layers and in different directions. They are like a bowl shaped container. The muscles cooperate to keep everything in place and form a floor for the organs in the abdomen, especially the bladder, prostate, seminal vesicles and rectum. There are two openings that allow for passage through the pelvic floor: the urethra in front of the perineum and the anus behind it. They have plenty of nerve endings and blood vessels that are sensitive to pressure. The pelvic floor muscles participate in the erection and get contractions during ejaculation. Many men are completely unaware of their pelvic floor muscles, where they are located and what they do.

Why train the pelvic floor muscles?

A strong pelvic floor is good for several reasons. The most important thing is to control the openings of bladder and anus, prevent incontinence, prevent or facilitate ejaculation, strengthen sexual performance and to support the internal organs. A muscle that is too weak causes the organs to become loose and hang down, and thus pressing against the perineum. A symptom of weak muscles can be incontinence or premature ejaculation. Many of the problems with the prostate or "chronic pelvic pain" are due to tense pelvic floor muscles. If you have removed your prostate, training to strengthen the area is even more important. According to Tao, the pelvic muscles also tonify all the other muscles in the body and strengthen your grounding in the body and connection with the earth. It is your base and is very important for your whole well-being. This is where your life force resides and due to Taoist and other eastern traditions it is the very foundation of your spiritual as well as your physical and sexual potential.

It is not only important to have strong pelvic floor muscles. Just as with all the other muscles in the body, it is equally important to be able to relax. Relaxation is needed for the blood to reach and oxygenate all the cells as well as for the nerves to work well. Both overly tense or too weak muscles decrease the blood flow, as well as the flow of Qi along the meridians in the pelvic floor. Over time, this can create imbalances that can eventually lead to ill health. By exercising the muscles of the pelvic floor, your strength, agility and sensitivity can develop. It will have a positive effect on your posture, breath and presence.

Some of the pelvic floor muscles are beyond your control. You can still influence the autonomic nervous system by releasing stress and relaxing the pelvic floor. That will affect the balance and harmonize the whole body.

Does it pay off to practice?

Muscles will wither and must be maintained. They quickly lose their strength without training, but are fortunately easy to train. If they are too tense you can, through awareness and exercise, teach them how to relax. There are few beginners who are able to isolate the correct squeezing, or relaxation though. You will need awareness of which muscles are concerned and knowledge of the best techniques. With the right guidance, most people can learn both quickly and easily. The first step is to get a better feel for the function of the pelvic floor and to find the muscles in yourself. Do the muscle test on page 133 before you begin. A complete exercise program should then include training of strength, speed and stamina as well as sensitivity and relaxation. Here we will train the sensitivity in the testicle breathing and strength and relaxation in connection to the squeezing exercises further along.

Which muscles is it?

The pelvic floor consists of three layers of muscle. The upper pelvic diaphragm, the urogenital diaphragm and at the bottom the bulbospongiosus and ischiocavernosus. The last two cover the root of the penis. Around the urethra, prostate and anus there are sphincters.

The pelvic diaphragm

These muscles run horizontally from the tailbone to the pubic bone and surround the urethra and anal duct. The diaphragm forms two upward reaching arches and is situated at the top of the pelvis, just below the prostate. The pelvic diaphragm is the largest muscle group with levator ani as its main muscle. Levator ani in turn, consists of three parts, of which the most significant is the pubococcygeus (PC-muscle) that lies adjacent to the prostate and anus. The other parts are puborectalis, iliococcygeus and even coccygeus belong here. Muscle tone of the pelvic diaphragm can be palpated through the anus.

The pelvic diaphragm assists the sphincters and is like the gatekeeper for the openings of the urethra and the anus. They lift the pelvic floor upward and slightly forward when contracted. It is primarily with this one that you can stop your urine and ejaculation. This muscle can also stimulate the prostate. With a well tonified pelvic diaphragm you will be better skilled to build and hold a bigger amount of orgasmic energy.

Urogenital diaphragm

Located in the front of the pelvis and crosses down below the pelvic diaphragm. It is triangular shaped with the base at the sit bones and top at the pubic bone. Sometimes called the perineal membrane and includes the deep and shallow transverse perineal muscles. They support the pelvic diaphragm and are important to fix the perineal body in the midline. The deep transverse perineal muscle permeates and stabilizes the root and the erection of the penis.

The muscles of the pelvic floor seen from underneath

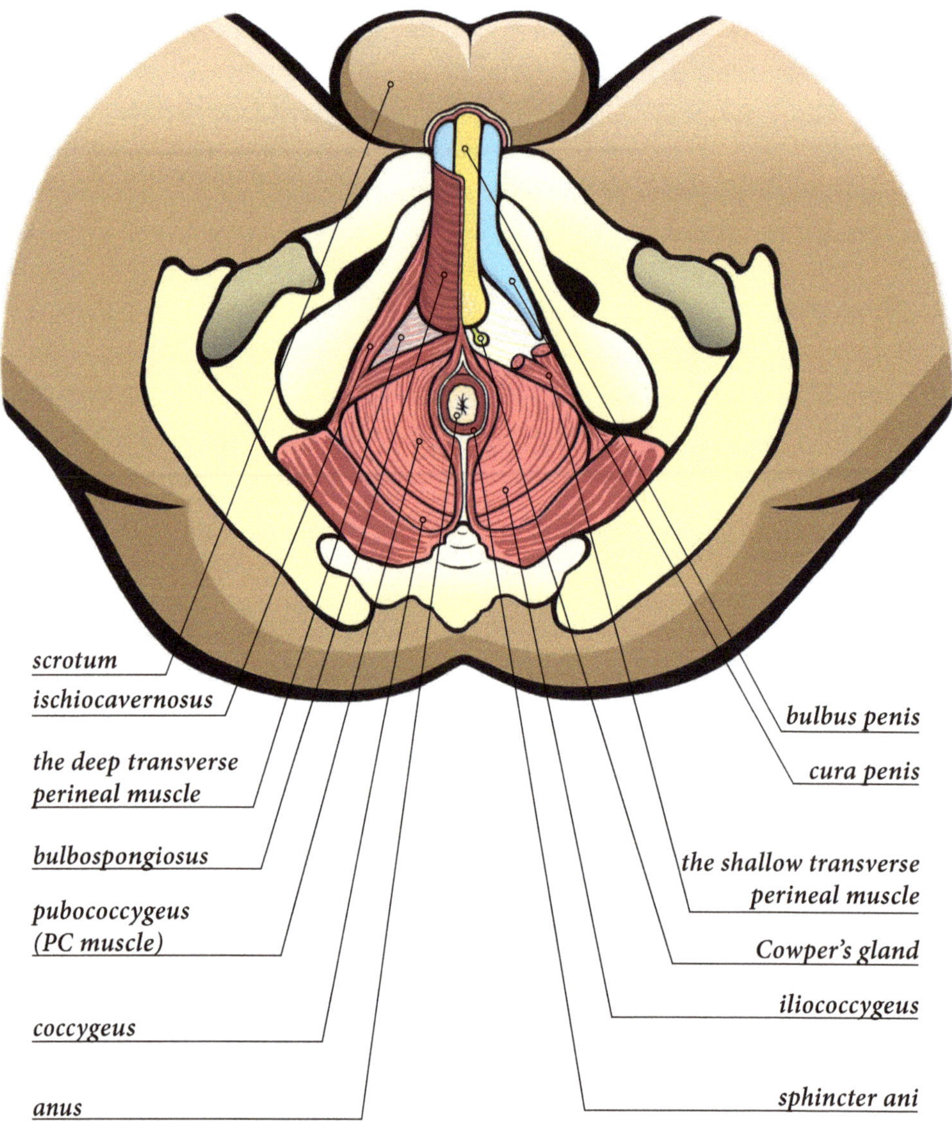

Bottom and sphincter muscles

At the bottom and in the front of the pelvic floor is the bulbospongiosus muscle and further out on the side the ischiocavernosus. They interweave with the root of the penis and connect to the perineal body. Both bulbospongiosus and ischiocavernosus can be contracted by will. They are easy to feel and play a significant role for the erection, expulsion of seminal fluid and sexual function.

An important thing for ejaculation is the contraction in bulbospongiosus. It pushes the contents of the urethra forward so that the pressure in the head of the penis increases, which enhances pleasure. Even the ischiocavernosus is contracted through ejaculation and contributes to the stiffness of the penis.

At the mouth of the prostate there is a striated sphincter, around the anus is the sphincter ani and around the urethral is the urethral sphincter. They are all under voluntary and not voluntary control.

Test your pelvic floor muscles

How do I know if I have an excessively weak or tight muscle? Note that a muscle that is too tight will become weak in the long run.

Test: Can you stop the beam by tightening when you pee?

If you can't stop the urine flow or find it difficult, you probably have weak muscles, or ignorance of how to use them. Also check in a mirror that the base of the penis moves up against the stomach and that the scrotum rises when you're squeezing.

The squeezing exercises and the numbers (amount, time etc.) that follow are just suggestions. Do fewer exercises or spend less time on them if they're too difficult, and increase as your strength increases. Regularity gives results. Notice your strengths and weaknesses.

- It's better to do a few dozen squeezes a day than none at all.

- Try to squeeze only with the pelvic floor muscles, relax your stomach, buttocks, thighs etc.

- There are many moments in everyday life that are great for training such as standing in line, on the bus, in front of the tv etc. No one can see what you're doing.

- Men with very weak pelvic floor muscles can start with as few as 10 squeezes a day that are accentuated for a 2-3 month period.

Guide exercise 12:

Time: 10-15 min

Purpose: Find the muscles 💙 Practice strength and relaxation 💙 Raise awareness of strength and sensitivity

Preparation: Basic position and warm-up exercises (standing, sitting or lying). Start by just squeezing. Find and feel the muscle. Notice how it feels and what happens when you're squeezing. Always relax after each squeeze.

1. Easy squeezing exercise

This simple squeezing exercise helps weak muscles become stronger and tense muscles relax. Can be done lying down (with your feet on the floor and knees bent and apart), sitting or standing.

- Squeeze for 5 seconds and relax for 5 seconds. It's just as important to relax as it is to squeeze. Do 10 squeezes, 3 times a day. Increase the number as time goes on.

- Goal: 30 squeezes per session, three times a day, five days a week until you are strong.

2. Get to know your pelvic floor muscles

Strength and relaxation:

- Squeeze on your inhale, and relax on your exhale. Repeat 10 times.

- Squeeze on your exhale and relax on your inhale. Repeat 10 times.

- Squeeze and hold for 10 seconds regardless of breathing, relax 10 seconds. Repeat 3 times.

Perseverance and speed:

- Squeeze 20 times as fast as you can. Use the muscles in the lower part of the pelvic floor.

- Squeeze as hard as you can and hold on your inhale. Use the muscles higher up in the pelvic floor. Repeat 3 times.

- Squeeze as hard as you can and hold on your exhale. Use the muscles higher up in the pelvic floor. Repeat 3 times.

Sensitivity:

- Squeeze in different ways; soft, hard, fast, slowly. Find which squeeze that activates the most feeling and energy for you. Do not mind your breathing, but feel the connection with your testicles, penis, prostate and anus.

The front of the pelvic floor

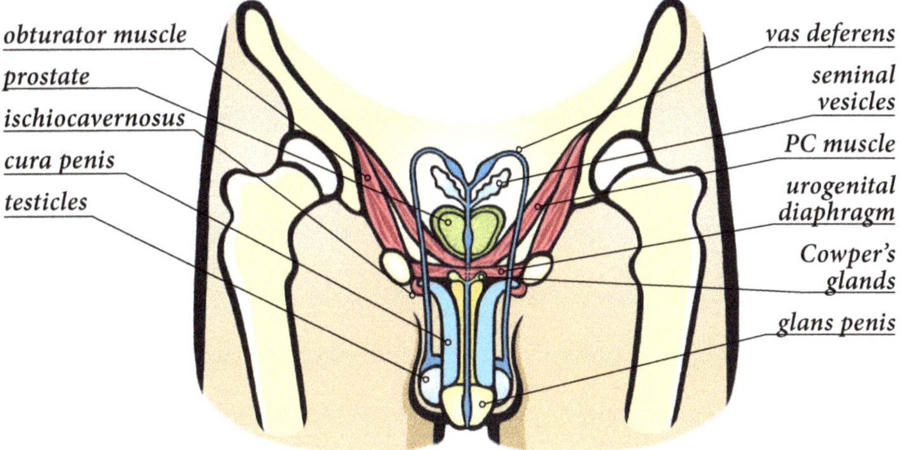

💧 Squeeze with a sucking feeling up through the penis and urethra, all the way up to your prostate. Like you want to drink and suck something up through your body. Activate all the muscle layers from the bottom to the pelvic diaphragm. Relax.

Awareness:

💧 Squeeze using the muscles and ligaments around the root of the penis, in the front of the pelvis. You should feel this just below the pubic bone.

💧 Squeeze using the muscles around the anus. You should feel this around your tailbone.

💧 Squeeze using the muscles at the perineum. You should feel this between the anus and the scrotum (almost all muscles meet here).

💧 Squeeze with the muscles on the left side, and then the right side. You should feel this by your sit bones. If you're standing you activate by lifting your heel a bit and press down with your toes. If you're lying or sitting you press each foot down into the floor. Will enable the urogenital diaphragm.

💧 Squeeze with the muscles at the bottom, the middle triangle, and the upper pelvic diaphragm one by one. Then imagine lifting them all together up into the body, as if you want to suck something up, and let go and relax.

EXERCISE 13:

Prostate massage

These exercises stimulate flow and circulation in and around the prostate. It promotes health as well as potency. Another advantage of regularly massaging your prostate is that you can detect tensions and indications of changes in size, elasticity or ache in the prostate. You access the prostate through the perineum or your anus. An additional benefit is that you help your pelvic floor and anus to free itself from unnecessary tension.

External prostate massage:

Time: 5 min

Purpose: Increase blood circulation ❤ Relaxation and awareness ❤ Increase health and potency

A simple and effective exercise that can be done every day. Do it lying on the floor or, for example, in bed before you get up or before you fall asleep.

Preparation: Horizontal warm-up and short inner smile.

1. Lie on your back with your knees towards the ceiling and the bottom of your feet against the floor. Spread your knees slightly.

2. Take some deep breaths and breathe all the way down into the pelvic floor, relax and rest inside yourself. Connect with your prostate. Breathe and smile towards your prostate. Feel how it loosens up and relaxes.

3. Massage the prostate through the perineum by stroking along the area from the anus to the root of the penis. Stroke with two fingers from each hand on each side of the area. About 1 minute.

4. Press using two fingers of each hand on each side of the area. Move gradually from the anus to the root of the penis and hold for 10 seconds in each place. Breathe down.

5. Place your hands above the pubic bone, the fingertips touch each other.

6. Press the middle fingers gently, backwards and downwards, toward the prostate. Gently massage with your fingers from side to side 10 times. You will feel where the prostate is.

7. Do the same a few centimeters up towards the navel. And again, until you reach the navel. Keep your attention inside and on the prostate.

8. Put your hands on Dan Tian, breathe down to the prostate and relax and just rest for a while.

Outer prostate massage

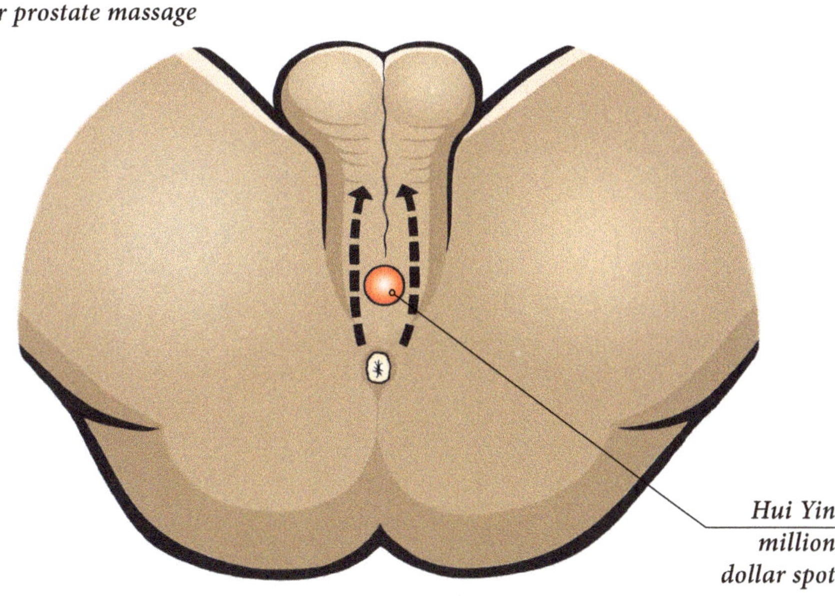

Stroke and gently press the perineum, from the anus to the root of the penis.

Outer prostate massage

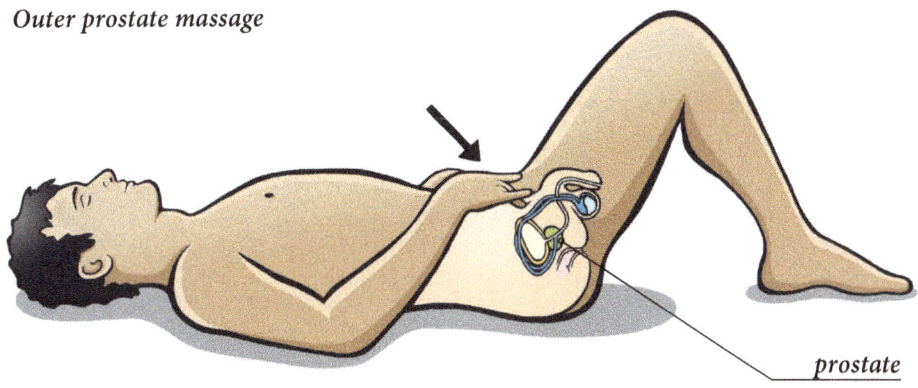

Massage the prostate through the lower abdomen.

Internal prostate massage

This massage is sometimes referred to as "milking" the prostate. By stimulating the prostate directly through the anus it may empty itself as a slow ejaculation. It is good to empty the prostate in this way if you don't want to ejaculate for some reason or if you don't have an active and healthy sex life at the moment. Many men experience an intense enjoyment during this stimulation, and it can lead to a different type of orgasm than from penis stimulation.

Time: 10 min

Purpose: Empty the prostate of fluid 💜 Stimulate blood flow and circulation 💜 Increase enjoyment and relaxation

Always massage softly and carefully. The prostate gland is much more sensitive and softer than the muscles. It should definitely not hurt and there should be no hard bumps or quick movements. Use plenty of oil or lubricant. The prostate is located approximately 2 inches in, on the front wall, toward the stomach.

Most people can just about access the prostate with a finger, use your index or middle finger. Therefore, it may also be useful to use a device (butt plug). There are special prostate stimulators that you can buy. If you use a device in the anal opening, it is best to have one with a clear stop, an anchor (and never use a device if you have acute prostatitis). It is important to perform the massage with care and sensitivity. Take care of your hygiene and wash yourself properly before and after. Gloves can be useful and convenient.

1. Sit or lie comfortably.

2. Take a few deep breaths, relax and rest into yourself.

3. Lubricate the anal opening and your finger.

4. Massage and loosen the anal opening.

5. Gently insert your finger (or device) into your anus by putting the finger (device) in the opening. Then squeeze a few times, with the finger in the opening, and during the relaxation the finger is slowly sliding in. As far as you can or feel comfortable with. Take your time. Never press using force.

6. Find and feel the prostate gland. Feels like a softer structure towards the stomach.

7. Keep a firm pressure on the prostate. Feel if it's sore, hard, soft, agile, mushy, insensitive, tense etc. Notice if it's relaxing and opening up. Notice also the status of the muscles around.

8. Do a little "come here" motion, towards the stomach, with your finger. Massage the sides, up and down the prostate. You may feel pleasure and ejaculate.

9. Remove your finger. Feel the flow of energy, relax and rest.

Inner prostate massage

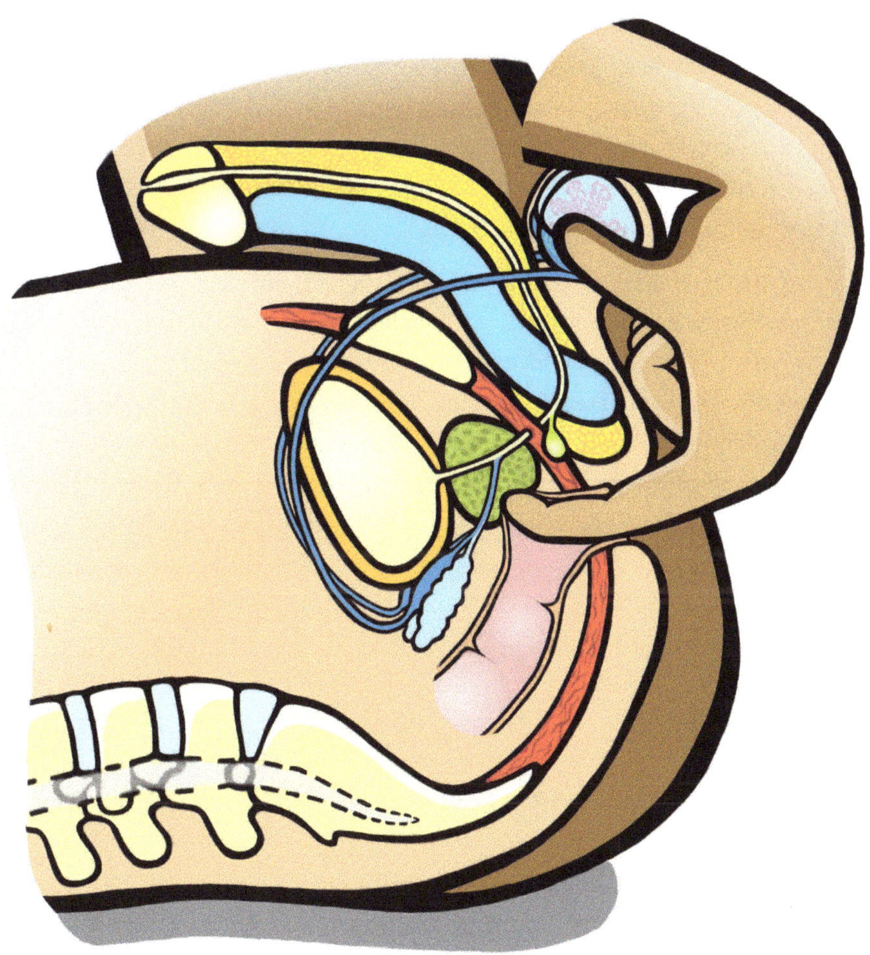

Massage the prostate through the anus. Feel the connection and increase your awareness about the prostate. Smile down and help it relax.

Withhold your ejaculation

The technique is to stop stimulating yourself before the ejaculation, just before the point of no return. Then relax and let the energy calm down and spread it through the body. Then repeat the same procedure again. This will change the habit of always being in a hurry and losing it. You will increase the level of orgasm you can hold without going over the edge. This allows you to expand your ability for pleasure and you can last longer. Finally you can get an orgasm without ejaculating.

According to a survey of multi-orgasmic men, they found that if a man learns to masturbate for 15-20 minutes without ejaculating, he has good conditions for making love as long as he wants with a partner. Tao calls masturbation self-development and sees it as an exercise in making use of the life-giving sexual energy. A quote from Mantak Chia: "Everyone wants to be sexy and therefore they train their biceps at the gym. Is it not more logical to train their genitals?"

The first step in controlling the arousal is breathing calmly and deeply, and relaxing even more when excitement increases. In addition, it helps having well-trained and flexible pelvic floor muscles which are also capable of relaxing. In the beginning you will probably have to stop several seconds before the point of no return. Use both your breathing and pelvic floor muscles to guide the energy upwards along the spine. If you're about to go over your limit, you squeeze with extra force. Exercise yourself to recognize the signals that come with the arousal and emission, such as breathing changes, a tingle in the root of your penis, contractions in the prostate and pelvic floor etc. This is something you practice to create a new natural pattern over time. Eventually you'll only need a clear intention to turn the flow.

Guide exercise 14:

Time: 10-20 min

Purpose: Stop the ejaculation ❤ Extend your pleasure ❤ Build orgasmic energy

Preparation: Lubricate the penis with nurturing natural oil. Feel free to do an inner smile before to strengthen self-acceptance and self-esteem. Let your consciousness merge with your penis and make it sensitive and receptive. Sit with a straight back and have the tip of your tongue against the palate during the exercise. The curious one may also, in the relaxation phase, focus on the pineal gland, in the middle of the head, while doing the soft squeezing. Then stay there until the arousal settles.

- Sit comfortably. Turn your attention inward, breathe deeply and relax.

- Connect with your penis and experience it from within.

- Masturbate and stroke yourself the way you like. Pay attention to your entire penis. Varying pressure, speed and grip.

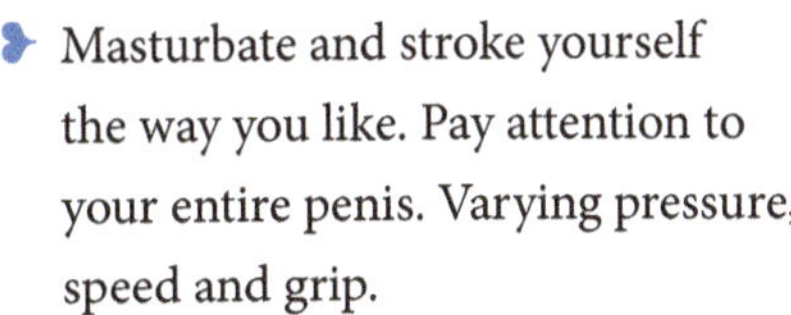

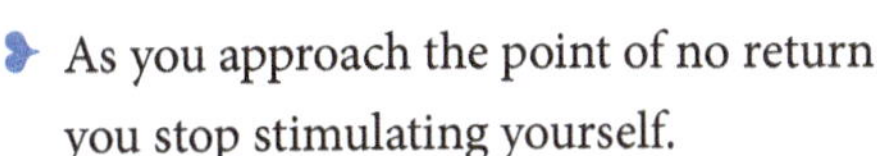

- As you approach the point of no return, you stop stimulating yourself.

- Then, breathe deeply and calmly and relax your body. Squeeze softly to guide the energy up along the spine, squeeze harder when needed. Guide the energy higher and higher up the body for each time. Relax even more and enjoy the energy. Let the energy cool down a little.

- Then continue to stroke yourself again closer to the point of no return, at least 3 times.

- Stop when you reached climax several times without ejaculating. Feel the energy rise in the body. Alternatively, allow yourself to go for it and come and spray fully.

- Enjoy the afterglow or you can guide the energy into the SC to transform the orgasmic energy into life energy.

When you're practicing with really aroused or orgasmic energy, which is very powerful, it is valuable to do energy exercises (standing tree, SC, charge your life energy, testicle breathing etc.). This is when the Jing energy transforms into Qi, life energy, and then to Shen, expansion of your consciousness, leading to cultivation of self-development, creativity and spirit connection.

To further boost your genital sense of self send love, appreciation and light to your penis. In the tantric tradition the male genital is called a "wand of light".

Tao prefers to withhold the ejaculation, but at the same time encourages being receptive to your natural flow and where the energy wants to go. Sense what feels best for you and be open to variations. Especially as you now know what is possible, and know the importance of exploring and experiencing different orgasms.

Ceremonies

A ceremony is a ritual, an act, with a symbolic meaning. It has a clear intention to guide the energy in a certain direction. Good timing for a ceremony to get support from the universal changers could be at full moon, equinox or solstice.

Purification ceremony

In this ceremony, you call on memories, experiences, thoughts, feelings and behaviors that you no longer need and which no longer benefit you. Ask for help to cleanse yourself and your genitalia.

- Call upon and perceive the emotions of the experiences and memories you want out of your system. Intensify the feeling and breathe in, bend your neck back and close your eyes.

- Bend your neck forward, open your eyes and exhale vigorously, and feel how all the emotions and memories you no longer need are leaving you. If you like, you can use voice and motions for full expression.

- Do the same again if more memories and feelings appear. When you're done, put your hands on Dan Tian and breathe calmly. Feel peace and stillness.

Then fill yourself with the new feelings and things that you want to let into your life. Let it come to you from the stillness.

Ceremony for your new dream

What do you want to create in your life? What is really important to you? What makes you happy and content? What are you passionate about, what new visions do you want to spark up? What do you want to feed and manifest? How do you want to live the rest of your life?

- Ask for a vision of new intentions, purposes and goals. What does your new dream look like?

- Then do some of the exercises (for example, testicle breathing that nourishes your creativity and life purpose) as usual.

- Let your new dream come to you in the yin phase after the practice. Do nothing, open yourself to the new, wait, be honest and true to the longing of your heart.

- Finish, say your thanks and pray for your dream to manifest.

Creative expression

These small ceremonies can be combined with a creative expression such as writing down your experiences or desires, painting them, making a collage or an altar with the new things you want to create in the future. Manifestation is about turning a future dream into reality in the present. A sense of that your wish has already been realized. You can also strengthen your dreams by sending your wish into the universe with your orgasm, the creative power itself.

Training tips

It's better to practice 15 minutes per day than one hour, one day, once a week. Your Qi grows by regularity and you break patterns by acquiring new habits. These are techniques that you practice over time rather than temporary experiences. Pick out a couple of exercises at a time to immerse yourself in. Gain experience by at least training three times a week for three months. Then you get an idea and feel for what an exercise can give you and if it works. A clear intention gives extra power in the exercise and increases your motivation. Don't forget that the yin phase is an important part of the exercise.

Example of exercise sequence

The basic training is the inner smile and the small circulation. Begin by balancing your emotions, cultivating self-acceptance and self-esteem and learning how to circulate energy. If you need to ground yourself then do the exercise with the tree. If you want to strengthen your sexual potency or if you have a weak pelvic floor then do squeezing exercises and testicle and prostate massages. If you want to increase your orgasmic ability, you focus on testicle breathing and work on holding back your ejaculation. Preparation is always the basic position (exercise 1) and preferably the warm-up exercises (exercise 2) and/or short inner smile (exercise 6). Finishing up is to collect the energy (exercise 3).

Suggestions for exercise combinations

The tree and the inner smile (exercise 4 + 5).

The inner smile and the small circulation (exercise 5 + 7).

Short inner smile and hormone shower (exercise 6 + 11).

Charge your life energy, testicle breathing and the small circulation (exercise 9 + 10 + 7).

Testicle massage and squeezing exercises (exercise 8 + 12).

Warm-up exercises lying down and external prostate massage (exercise 2 + 13).

Magic tools

Hope you have profited from reading this book and have been inspired to take on the exercises. You can view all exercises as magic tools or as keys to help you even further on your path through life. In the beginning, you guide your energy, but eventually you will learn to follow your natural current. Mastering a technique is not the most important thing, but to master yourself and find as much space for self-reflection and rest you need in everyday life. A place to which you can return and bring vitality, happiness and wisdom. Keep in mind that you are unique and valuable and can choose to say yes to cultivating your masculine power and radiance.

Good luck with your practice and the development of your full potential!

REFERENCES

Books

Andersson, Iréne (2011): *Kvinnans Tao: Vägen till glädje, njutning och livsenergi!* [Create Health with Your Sexual Energy: The Tao approach to womens well-being]. Stockholm: Procreative AB.

Chang, Stephen T. (1992): *The Tao of sexology: The Book of infinite wisdom.* Tao publ.

Chia, Mantak (2003): *Karsai Nei Tsang: Genital therapeutic cleansing massage.* Chiang Mai: North star trust.

Chia, Mantak et al. (2005): *The Multi-orgasmic couple: Sexual secrets every couple should know.* San Francisco: HarperOne.

Chia, Mantak & Winn, Michael (1984): *Taoist secrets of love: Cultivating male sexual energy.* Santa Fe: Aurora press.

Deida, David (2002): *Finding God through sex: Awakening the one of spirit through the two of flesh.* Louisville: Sounds True.

Lai, Hsi (2002): *The sexual teachings of the jade dragon: Taoist methods for male sexual revitalization.* Vermont: Destiny Books.

Richardson, Diana (2008): *The heart of tantric sex.* New Alresford: John Hunt Publishing.

Richardson, Diana and Richardson, Michael (2010): *Tantric sex for men: Making love a meditation.* Toronto: Destiny books.

Books about sexuality

Charles, Amara (2005): *Conscious sexual agreements.* Phoenix: Nourishing arts.

Charles, Amara (2011): *The sexual practices of Quodoushka.* Rochester: Destiny Books.

Drevstam, Malin (2010): *Tidig utlösning: orsaker, konsekvenser och behandlingar av prematur ejakulation.* [Early ejaculation: Causes, consequences and treatments of premature ejaculation]. Stockholm: Gothia förlag.

Geels A. & Roos L. (red.).(2010). *Sex – för guds skull: Sexualitet och erotik i världens religioner.* [*Sex - for God's sake: Sexuality and eroticism in the world's religions*]. Lund: Studentlitteratur.

Hulter, Birgitta (2004): *Sexualitet och hälsa.* [*Sex and health*]. Lund: Studentlitteratur.

Komisaruk, Barry R. M.fl. (2002): *The Science of orgasm.* Baltimore: The Johns Hopkins University Press.

Löfgren-Mårtenson, Lotta (2013): *Sexualitet.* [*Sexuality*] Malmö: Liber.

Sexologi: [*Sexology*] (2010):Under red. av P.O. Lundberg. Stockholm: Liber.

Sister Sofie o.p. Hamring (2011): *Till man och kvinna skapade han dem: En introduktion till kroppens teologi.* [*Created to man and woman by Him: An introduction to the theology of the body*]. Skellefteå: Artos.

Books about Qigong

Cohen, Kenneth S. (1999): *The way of Qigong: The art and science of Chinese energy healing.* New York: Ballantine Books.

Mitchell, Damo (2002): *Daoist Nei Gong: The philosophical art of change.* London: Singing dragon.

Skarpste-Malmqvist, Ruta (2007): *Dokument Qigong: Kraftfull väg till självläkning och ökad livskvalité:* Bakgrund, effekter och forskningsresultat. [*Document Qigong: Powerful Approach to Self-Health and Increased Life Quality:* Background, Effects and Research Results]. Fritsla, Förlagstryckeriet Vinterleken.

Tze, Yuan (2010): *Voyage to the shore: An invitation to enhance your health and develop your life:* Part 2. Wellington: Yuan Tze center.

Other Books

Billing, Pelle (2012): *Jämställdhetsbluffen.*[*Equality bluff*]. Stockholm: Billing.

Brizendine, Louann (2008): *The female brain.* New York: Bantam Books.

Childre, Doc et al. (1999): *The Hearthmath solution.* San Francisco: Harper

Frank, Lone (2009): Mindfield: *How brain science is changing our world.* London: Oneworld Publ.

Haug, E et al.(1993): *Människans fysiologi.* [*Human physiology*]. Stockholm: Liber utbildning: Universitetsförlaget.

Mares, Théun (1999): *The Toltec teachings:* Volume III. 3rd ed. Athens: Renascent Legacy Press.

Matus, Lujan (2005): *The art of stalking parallell perception: The living tapestry of Lujan Matus*. UK: Trafford publ.

Olsson, Anders (2012): *Medveten andning: Grunden för hälsa, energi och harmoni.* [*Consious breathing: The base for health, energy and harmony*]. Sorena.

Rosin, Hanna (2013): *The end of man: And the rise of women.* Stockholm: Riverhead books..

Röhlander, Olof (2011): *Det blir alltid som man tänkt sig: handbok i mental styrketräning.* [*It always becomes as you think: a manual in mental strength training*]. Stockholm: Månpocket.

Wise, David and Andersson, Rodney (2012): *A Headache in the pelvis: The Wise-Anderson Protocol for healing pelvic pain.* New York: Harmony books.

Articles

Hansson, Catharina (1999): *Hitta P-punkten med erotisk Kung Fu.* [*Find the P-spot with erotic Kung Fu*] Fitness Man, nr 3, s 65-68.

Simeonova, Zwetanka: *Andropaus* (2001): *Det manliga klimakteriet.* [*The male menopause*]. Medikament, nr 4, s 104-107.

Web references:

Droppe, Adam (2010): Konstitueringen av ett vetenskapligt objekt: Exemplet – det manliga klimakteriet. [The constitution of a scientific object: The example – the male menopause]. www.diva-portal.org/smash/get/diva2:318919/FULLTEXT01.pdf

Frank, P. (1996). Här har du din nya kärlekszon.[Here is your new love-zon]. From: home.swipnet.se/~w-59099/ samlevn/Apunkt.htm

Grönberg, Henrik: Vem får prostatacancer? [Who gets prostate cancer?]. www.medfak.umu.se/digitalAssets/2/2801_prostata_2gronberg.pdf

Hedelin, Hans : Kronisk abakteriell prostatit/kroniskt bäckensmärtsyndrom. [Chronic abnormal prostatitis/chronic pelvic pain syndrome]. www.lakartidningen.se/store/articlepdf/1/14032/LKT1012s837_839.pdf

Lerner, Tomas: Porrimpotens: [Adult impotence].Verkligheten inte tillräckligt upphetsande. www.dn.se/insidan/verkligheten-inte-tillrackligt-upphetsande/Pdf

Prostataliknande besvär [Pains possibly related to prostatitis]. www.praktiskmedicin.se/sjukdomar/prostatitliknande-besvar-kronisk-abakteriell/

RFSU: Vuxna behöver sexualupplysning. [Adults need sexual instruction] www.familjeliv.se/Foralder/1.1983222

INDEX

LIST OF ILLUSTRATIONS

THANK YOU!

Thank's to my teachers and inspirers!

I would like to honor and thank some of the most significant teachers to me, who contributed in various ways by sharing their knowledge and wisdom.

💙 Andrew Fretwell 💙 www.wuji-gong.org

Andrew who travels worldwide teaching Wuji Gong is inspiring humanity to awaken self-love by grounding and crystalizing the essence of self (SOUL) and integrating it within the body/mind.

Andrew is also a great bodyworker and the founder of The OFT - Original Feeling Touch – an innovative healing modality. He also teaches Taoist alchemy as well as Taoist sexual practice. Universal Tao senior instructor.

💙 David Verdesi 💙 www.davidverdesi.com

David has devoted his life to the human potential, primarily through his exploration of Taoism, Tantra and shamanism. He has a rich and profound knowledge of Qigong and Taoism and its theory, science and training. A true source of inspiration of self-knowledge and pointing out the nature of the human potential.

💙 Mantak Chia 💙 www.universal-Tao.com

Master Chia is a knowledgeable and practical teacher who has summarized the Taoist wisdom from various teachers and shared it through many books and taught it all over the world. He is the one who has brought several of the Taoists Sexual Qigong exercises to the West and calls his system of methods Universal Tao.

❤ **Yuan Tze** ❤ www.yuantzecenter.com

Yuan Tze is a very inspiring Qigong master who came regularly to Sweden. He has a passion for healing, the development of human consciousness and a healthy lifestyle in harmony with mother earth. He has also formulated his insights into several books.

❤ **Åsa Kullberg** ❤ www.asakullberg.com

Åsa teaches with great passion and amazing clarity shamanic sexual wisdom, which is a ceremonial process to reconnect and remember the naturalness of who you are as a sexual human being. The teachings are based in a shamanic tradition, Quodoushka, from the Sweet Medicine Sundance Path. It also includes Shamanic Body Dearmoring, a two-week process that frees and expands the overall life force energy and stimulates vital health and happiness.

Thank's to others

I would like to thank Lisa Larsson for her tireless work, resulting in all the amazing illustrations. Johan Badh for doing the basic translation and then Deborah Sundahl for invaluable feedback on the text, as well as Allan Stein and Cosma Gills. For excellent proofreading I would like to thank Kicki Pallin and Lucas Serby and then Ann-Sofie Hammarström Östergren for exemplary and professional work with the cover and layout. Special thanks to Andrew Kenneth Fretwell for inspiration and quotes, Björn Westin for specialist review and Ann-Margret Kälfors for help with the Swedish text. Others I want to mention with thankfulness is Jens Hansen, Jonas Karlström, Björn Fernström and Toini Pettersson, as well as all of you who have given feedback or supported this project. Thank you all!

Further information

❤ www.pelvicfloorawareness.com & www.bodycoach.nu
❤ info@bodycoach.nu

Other books published in English by Irene Andersson:
❤ Create Health with Your Sexual Energy: The Tao Approach to Women's Well-Being

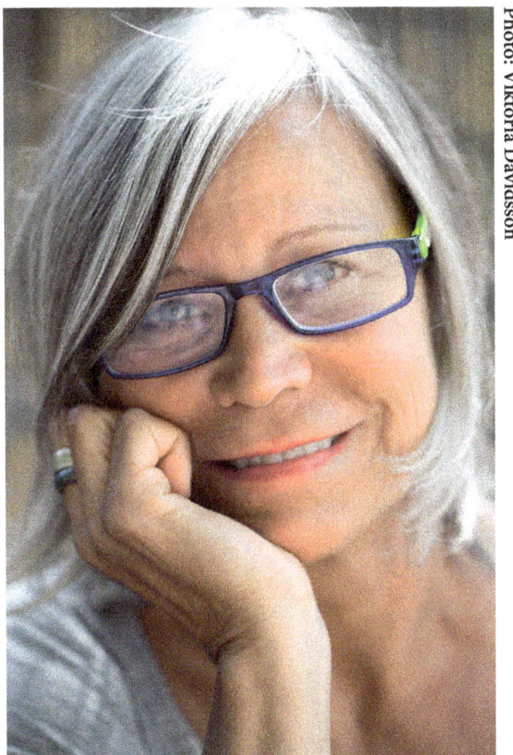

About Iréne Andersson

Iréne Andersson is from Sweden and has over 25 years of exploration and learning in different traditions and alternative methods, resulting in a unique combination of knowledge, experience and tools. Her specialty is Taoist sexual practice with focus on the pelvic floor and sexual health. She combines modern research with wisdom from different traditions of thought that has a holistic view. Iréne is a certified Qigong instructor since 1998 and has spent a lot of time with Taoist teachers in different countries, and also studied Tantra and shamanism as well as psychological methods and school medicine. Iréne is passionate about sharing her knowledge of our bodies and erotic potential. In a clinical setting, she offers pelvic floor treatment and bodywork, and gives trainings, workshops and lectures in pelvic floor awareness, sexual health and Taoist sexual practice.

www.pelvicfloorawareness.com

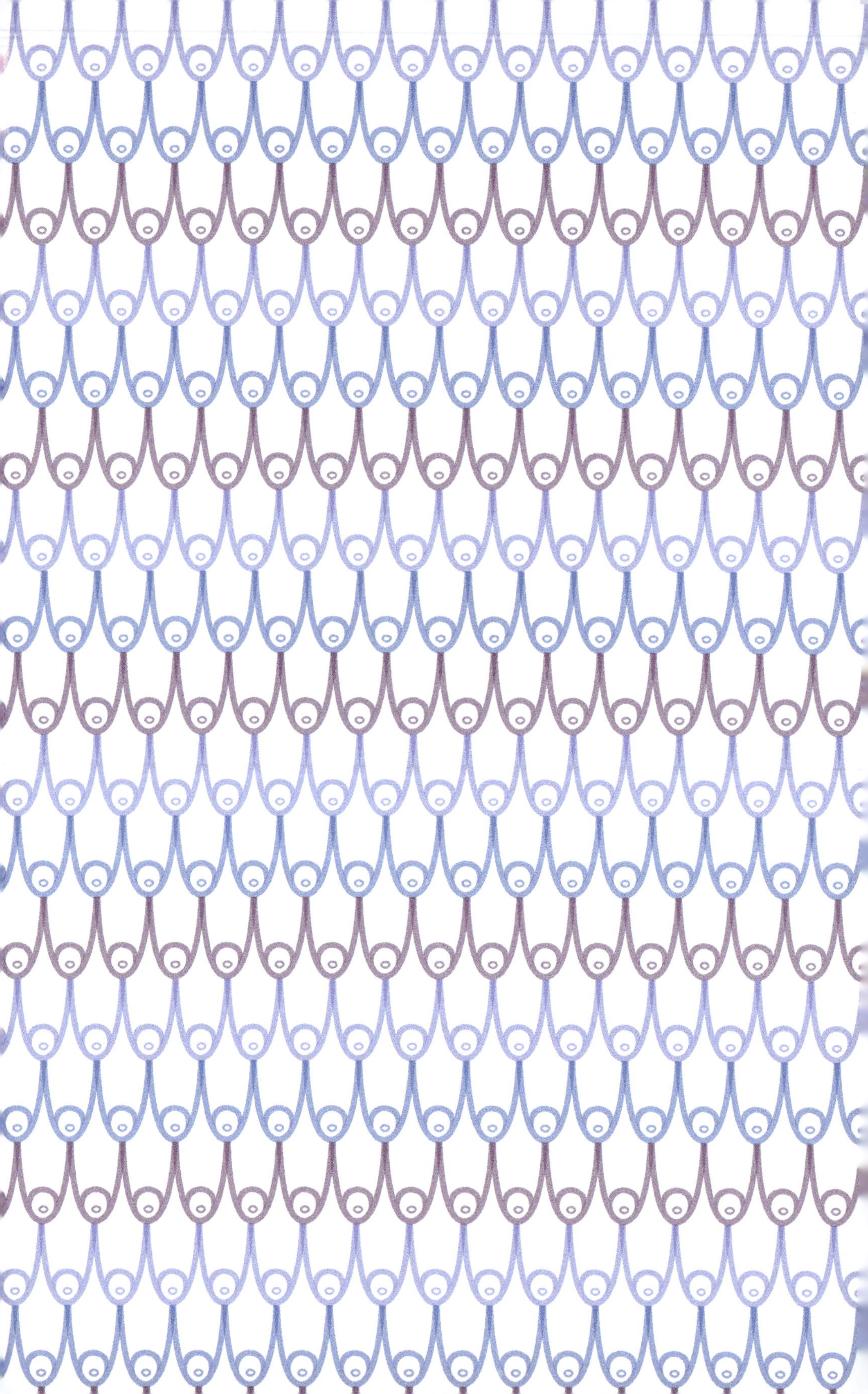

www.ingramcontent.com/pod-product-compliance
Lightning Source LLC
LaVergne TN
LVHW051109180726
843512LV00011B/771